The Much Bet

The Much Better You

Your wellbeing and mental health sorted

Dr Romano Giorgi

The Much Better You.
Copyright © 2023 by Dr Romano Giorgi.
All rights reserved.
TheMuchBetterYou.com
London, UK.
Cover concept by Sila and Romano.
Cover artwork by Katarina.
Edited by Sila.
Copy-edited by Sam.
ISBN: 9798366831239

£1 of this author's profits per copy of this book sold will go to **MIND**: The mental health charity that makes sure no one has to face a mental health problem alone.

Please visit mind.org.uk, see what they're about plus make a further donation.

For Dad

Contents:

	Page:
Foreword	13
Introduction	21
Chapter 1: First, let's get our house in order	25
1. Invest in your sleep	28
2. Declutter your life	31
3. Beware: Digital dementia	36
4. Say "no" more	40
Chapter 2: Know thy self	47
5. Keep your promises	50
6. Be yourself	55
7. Don't compare yourself to others	61
8. Limit your limiting beliefs	66
9. Embrace criticism	74
10. Be responsible	78
Chapter 3: Are you positive?	89
11. Shift your perspective	94
12. Watch your self-talk	100
13. Don't be a victim	105
14. Practice gratitude	108

15.	Focus on the positive	116

Chapter 4: What actually matters?		125
16.	Live with the end in mind	128
17.	Find your Why	132
18.	Look at the bigger picture	137

Chapter 5: Connection, connection, connection		143
19.	Be genuinely appreciative of others	146
20.	Pause, aim, fire	151
21.	Remember names	156
22.	Learn to listen	161
23.	Don't preach	169
24.	Love is a verb	174
25.	Love thy enemies	179

Chapter 6: Accept reality		187
26.	Accept that which you cannot control	189
27.	Manage adversity	194
28.	Reframe with humour	201

Summary:	205

Chapter 7: Tick Tock		211
29.	Live in the Now	213

30. Use your time well	219
Outro:	225
Closing Thought:	229
Acknowledgements:	233
Resources:	237

The Much Better You

Your wellbeing and mental health sorted

Foreword:

I once passed a Labrador having a poo in a park while simultaneously being humped by a miniature poodle. As I unconvincingly tried not to look on, I realised at that moment we are all basically just animals with similar needs and instincts.

The problem with us humans, though, is that we also have this pesky thing known as 'self-awareness' going on, some of us more than others. While self-awareness usefully enables us to reflect and challenge the validity of our thoughts, which is pretty damn useful and profound, it also causes us to overthink certain things, thus creating stress, anxiety and a raft of other issues.

This book is not for constipated Labradors or horny poodles, miniature or otherwise; it is for you and all the non-serving complexities that you bring with you.

I've never written a proper book before, though, so please bear with. Well, technically, I once wrote a PhD thesis which I recently tried to re-read, but I must confess I understood none of it. I also wrote a comedy-horror movie screenplay called 'Blood Moon', but the less said about that the better!

These 'literary events' feel so long ago now that I can barely recognise myself in them. Sure, I wrote them, but a lot has changed in me (and the planet) since then, so what I'm writing about now is a totally different kettle of fish.

Like many, I set out on this journey:

Born → curiosity → study → job(s) → mortgage → family → bigger mortgage → acquiesce → retire → die.

And like many, I didn't question 'The System' (or I may have thought I did, like most young rebels, but I was probably looking at an incomplete rendition of it). The problem was, however, that I didn't find my studies or my jobs to be especially fulfilling. They were merely a means to achieve things that, mostly, were themselves not especially fulfilling either. I had become one of society's automatons. And for what? A nicer car and a home with a mortgage on it that would keep me working until I was at least sixty-five.

The following question began to no longer sit comfortably with me:

If one should strive 'to live each day as if it were their last', then why am I spending at least 46 weeks of my 52-week year working long hours in a job that doesn't fulfil me?

It is only in the last few years that I have fully realised how important personal growth and continuous self-actualisation are to real fulfilment, and how important fulfilment is to wellbeing. Now I have a clearer sense of purpose, a stronger passion that drives me, and part of that passion is to help others along a similar sort of journey to improved living to the one I've been (and am!) on.

* * *

The Much Better You has been about four years in the making. If you listened to season 1 of my podcast, *The 3 in 15 Podcast*, upon which much of this book is based, you'll know that this book was mostly born out of multiple Covid-19 lockdowns that saw me spending much more time at home than I was used to. I soon realised that I had a choice on what I was going to be at the other side of lockdown: fit or fat, inspired or stagnant.

For the first time in my whole life, I put time, effort and structure into bettering myself in a way that would also serve others. I won't go into the specifics here, but I undertook a number of counselling, mental health and personal development training courses and consumed a truckload of complementary books.

Some of the most foundational and life-bettering self-improvement books out there are pretty damn amazing. We should feel so fortunate to benefit from the collective wisdom of thousands of incredible lifetimes. However, I must confess that some of these books are hard work because their content can be dense, academic and occasionally laden with technicalities. Had it not been for my being stuck at home, I may have not persevered with some. There's plenty of good stuff in them all though. The key is to keep an open mind and keep going.

Conversely, I also found that some books I came across were too spiritual to be taken seriously or, while being much easier to follow and better designed to be accessible for the layperson, their content was often too thin to enable one to get stuck into the principles in a practical and effective way.

Yes, you've guessed it: I'm building up to the angle that makes this book different (and much better...) ***The Much Better You*** takes many of the foundational principles that I learned throughout this journey and packages them up in a way that anyone can wrap their chops around.

I have added to the mix a generous sprinkling of true stories that will better enable the principles to pop from their pages. Someone, somewhere, once said words to the effect of:

"*The more personal the stories, the more universal their appeal*"

Why create a personal growth book that not everyone can relate to, understand or use? I want this book to help you to improve your life while being as easy to grasp as possible. If you can floss, you can follow this book.

I have grouped principles together into chapters that follow a common thread and will enable you to dip in and out of this book as and when you please. I have also sought to introduce some light-heartedness and humour into the mix to bear some of the burden of the heavier principles, while simultaneously keeping your interest piqued and your receptors sharp!

I want this book to lead you to reflect on the following statements and perhaps even conclude that they are not that far-flung but true:

The world owes you nothing.

Your perception of reality is not reality.

How you see the problem is the problem.

Thoughts are just thoughts.

You are not your past, and your past is not your future.

Gratitude will improve any aspect of your life.

Most of us are sleep-walking through our lives.

You are responsible for everything that is right or wrong with your life.

Where you are now results from all the decisions YOU have taken throughout your life.

Most of us are incapable of active listening.

Saying 'no' is one of the best things you can do to improve your mental health.

You are only ever one decision away from changing your life for the better.

Fear kills more dreams than failure does.

True fulfilment comes from being of service to others.

Some principles in this book are based on my own experiences and that what may resonate for me may not necessarily translate over into your own life in the same way. I ask only that you remain open-minded, not least of all because this book holds no punches. What would be the point of that?

* * *

Anyway, no one likes a waffly foreword so I will offer three further quickies before we dive right in.

First, none of the principles in this book are given as advice; they are merely designed to challenge your thinking, your status quo. It is up to you whether you apply them to your life or not. I learnt this 'never give advice' rule during a person-centred counselling course I undertook. If your friend is in an abusive relationship, for instance, it is much better to ask them what advice they would give someone else in their position than telling them to dump their partner (and risk them resenting you for it afterwards).

The second fundamental thing that this course taught me is that self-reflection and objective feedback from others is always the first step in any worthwhile endeavour. How, for instance, can you counsel someone else when you are not willing to be counselled yourself?

And finally, we ALL know the health benefits of a balanced diet and of regular exercise. It's simple really. Yet many of us won't eat well or go to the gym regularly.

The same applies to this book. While the principles and their benefits are clear cut and simple, not everyone will choose to commit to them because *their desire to improve their mental health or their desire to live a happier and more fulfilling life will be smaller than their desire to remain the same.* This may be down to fear of change or the momentum of procrastination for instance.[1]

Two people dear to me are each a case in point with this kind of thing. They both have mental health issues, and they live unfulfilled lives, BUT they will fight for their limitations passionately and sometimes even aggressively. I will go a little bit more into this later on, but the reason I bring them up here is that they are one of the main driving forces behind this book. While I don't expect them to read it anytime soon, I am determined to help them absorb the gold dust life hacks that lie within its pages.

I was also like them, in many respects, not too long ago, but I did

---

[1] But that's okay, this book will always be here and waiting for them should they decide to shake it up sometime!

something about it and improved my life dramatically by applying the contents of this book to my own life.

I'm still a work in progress.

Aren't we all?

Enjoy :)

Introduction:

No matter what life throws at you, be it a lottery win, financial dire straits or losing a loved one, it is *how you choose to respond* to these events that will determine whether you sink or swim, grow stronger or weaker, move forward or stay unhealthily anchored to the past. It is *how you choose to respond* to these events that will determine your outcomes. And this requires you to take full responsibility for yourself:

Responsible = Response + Able

Most of us crave fulfilment, happiness and connection; yet many of us will not take the steps necessary to achieve these outcomes. Instead, we will live life on autopilot. We get up, we go to a job that may or may not fill us with joy, we come home, we have dinner, we slump in front of the TV to watch Netflix and the daily news (invariably about negative things); then with all those depressing images still fresh in our brains, we go to bed, and the next day we repeat and so on and so forth. And let us not forget all the in-between moments, often hours on any day, looking at our smartphones, reacting to the agendas of others via emails, WhatsApp messages or the endless barrage of social media posts.

Whether you consider these things to be necessities or not,[2] it may be your past conditioning or limiting beliefs that tell you that, even though your job (you know, that thing that takes up half your life and

---
[2] I'm sure your 9 to 5 job is a necessity for instance.

most of your best years) may not fulfil you, you HAVE to do it anyway.

If you dread Monday mornings and only live for weekends or holidays, something may well be missing.

Don't allow your salary to buy your dreams from you.

* * *

We are all pre-conditioned to think or act in particular ways: early on, perhaps it's our parents, siblings or schools; later on, it's our peer groups, social circles and the media that will influence us. For instance, our sense of expression, joy, adventure and fun is often admonished out of us by our parents when we are young, in their well-intentioned effort to get us to behave in a way that is "normal" and "socially acceptable" with pernicious expressions such as "children should be seen but not heard." While this may pay dividends at a funeral, as Spike Milligan[3] once observed, most of us will lose our natural sense of humour, awe, excitement, curiosity and even creativity when we become adults.

Or perhaps there were some life events, either within or beyond our control, that now cause us to think or react in particular ways to particular triggers. This means that, more often than not, our thoughts and beliefs won't be objective and so may well not be serving us. These deeply-held, and often subconscious, beliefs may

---

[3] Legendary comedian and writer.

tell you that you're not smart enough or that you're too old to change jobs; or just another few years and that mortgage will get paid off, and then your real fulfilled life begins.

NEWSFLASH: *If it hasn't already, your fulfilled life should begin NOW.*

As long as you're not trying to defy the laws of physics or nature, you can do whatever you choose to do.

* * *

This book is packed with life hacks that, should you act upon them, will help to transform your life for **The Much Better You.** "**Your wellbeing and mental health sorted**" (this book's subtitle) is a bold claim, but I stand by it because many people whose teachings I am passing on to you are recognised leaders in their field and have studied and developed effective strategies to living an improved life. My own specific contributions, albeit heavily researched, are based on my own experiences of what works for me and those around me. I am sure they can work for you too.

When I told him I would start cycling to work in London, a wise friend once told me: *"When commuting on your bike, never be in a rush or else you are sure to come unstuck."*

Well, the same applies to you and this book. Even though it's packed with potentially life-changing principles, you don't have to try to do everything at once like some crash diet. Instead, take your time to learn, reflect and then apply in a steady and sustainable manner those principles you believe will work for you. You need not do them all, you know. Just start by doing something!

The list of life principles I'm presenting you with here isn't exhaustive. But the ones included are amongst the most fundamental and pertinent to the world these days. Pretty much every personal growth or wellbeing podcast that I have listened to recently (and believe me, I listen to many) cites variations on these principles that assure me that the content of this book is both up-to-date and powerful.

* * *

Human quirkiness is a highly complex thing. Each of us is a marvellous mystery, spun out of random circumstances, occurrences and genetic codes. It is amazing that the principles we are about to cover are such powerful tools, and so broadly applicable, that they somehow transcend these complexities and differences. That they are somehow so... human.

The Much Better You begins here...

CHAPTER 1

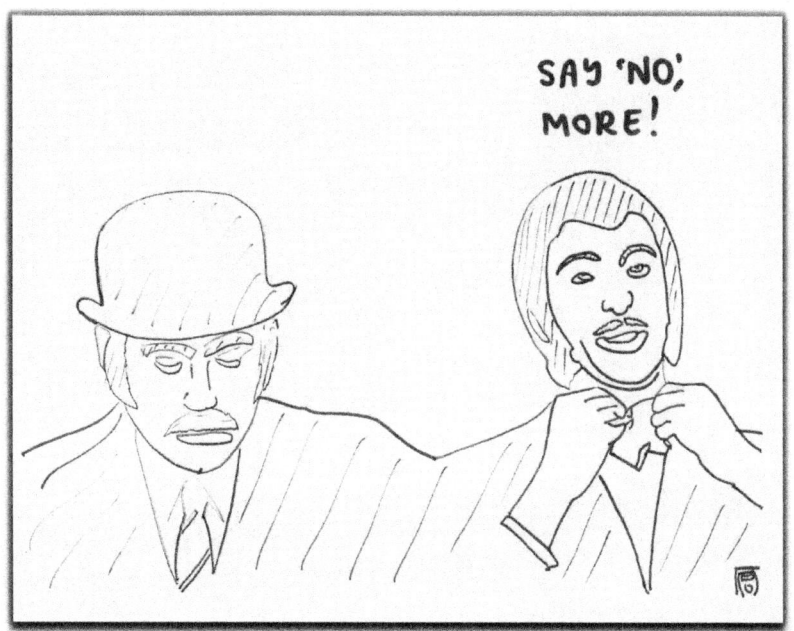

CHAPTER 1

First, let's get our house in order

This chapter describes some pretty foundational principles that will set the scene for the rest of this book but, much more importantly, will transform your life for the better should you choose to apply them yourself or share them with the people that matter the most to you.

Nothing in this chapter should surprise you, which may then beg the question: Why aren't you striving to do all these things?

Unlike later in this book (where I will), I'm not trying to give you a hard time here. Hell, I'm still struggling to follow some of these principles myself. For instance, I still use my smartphone way too much and don't always keep my sleeping hours consistent. The key thing is that when I adhere to these principles, everything gets much better for me. And it'll get much better for you too.

Let's get stuck in...

* * *

1. Invest in your sleep:

"The best bridge between despair and hope is a good night's sleep"
– E. Joseph Cossman, inventor and author.

Sleep is the foundation upon which the other principles in this book are based. Besides, it crosses over to all areas of our health, so let's start with this.

According to sleep scientist Professor Matthew Walker, sleep is your "life-support system and mother nature's best effort yet at immortality". Walker references in his interviews and excellent TED talks significant studies that demonstrate the alarmingly bad things that happen to you, both cognitively and physiologically, when you don't get enough sleep. Without wishing to give you nightmares (no pun intended), check out these four nasties from his horror list:

- There is a global sleep experiment that takes place twice a year. This is known as daylight saving hours, where in spring we lose an hour and in autumn we gain an hour. According to studies[4], when we lose an hour of sleep in spring, the next day, heart attack rates increase across the globe by 24%. But when we gain an hour in autumn, we see a 21% reduction in heart attacks. This same profile is approximately reflected in the rates of road traffic accidents and even suicides. Pretty shocking.

---

[4] Sandhu A, Seth M, Gurm HS. Daylight savings time and myocardial infarction. Open Heart 2014; 1;e000019.doi:10.1136/openhrt-2013-000019

- Sleep deprivation is well known to be linked to cardiovascular disease, neurological diseases such as dementia, premature ageing and cancer. The World Health Organisation (WHO) (I said: The World Health Organisation!) has listed all forms of night shift work as a carcinogen!

- There is no major psychiatric condition in which sleep is normal.

- Men who regularly sleep 5 hours a night have testicles significantly smaller than men who sleep 7 hours or more[5].

Essentially there is not one part of our physiological or neurological health not negatively affected by poor sleep.

So, what can we do to address this?

Here are easy wins that Walker recommends for improved sleep:

- Adults should get somewhere between 7 and 9 hours sleep a night.

- Go to bed at the same time every night and get up at the same time every morning, regardless of weekdays or weekends, because we are programmed to be creatures of habit. According to clinical psychologist and author, Professor Jordan Peterson, many of his

---

[5] I bet this last one caught you unaware unless you already don't sleep and have small bollocks.

clients' anxiety levels were reduced to subclinical levels merely because they slept on a predictable level.

- Sleep at a slightly lower temperature of 65 degrees Fahrenheit, or a little over 18 degrees Celsius, as dropping your body's core temperature by 1 degree Celsius helps you sleep more quickly, better and for longer. Turn the thermostat down at night and fewer blankets, not more!

- Darkness is king. Sleep in a dark room by using blackout blinds or eye masks, for instance. Plus, an hour or so before going to bed, try dimming the lights as this will help you to get sleepy. And please KEEP AWAY from bloody smartphones[6], tablets or bright computer screens as the associated 'blue light' can inhibit the production of the "sleep hormone", melatonin.

- Try to minimise caffeine and alcohol consumption, particularly closer to bedtime.

- Avoid napping during the day.

And finally...

- If you can't sleep at night when you go to bed, get out of bed and do something in another room instead until you feel sleepy again as otherwise your mind will make an unhealthy association between

---

[6] WARNING: I give smartphones a very hard time in this book.

lack of sleep and your bed. This also means not watching TV[7] or eating dinner in bed, you lazy shit.

Invest in your sleep.

2. Declutter your life:

"Clutter is anything that gets between you and the life that you want to be living" - Peter Walsh, professional organizer (yes, that's a job)

As I pull this book together, there's a crazy war unfolding in Ukraine. And so, a few weeks ago, I wanted to donate clothes and shoes to displaced Ukrainian refugees. Yes, I'm a lovely person. I went through my clothes drawers and wardrobe and was struck by three 'Hows':

- How much clutter there was. Clutter being defined here as a state of untidy, busy disorder, which by the way, can apply to both physical items and to 'emotional baggage' states;

- How much crap I owned that I had forgotten about and hadn't worn in several years; and

- How emotionally attached I was to these things.

---

[7] Various studies have shown that couples that have TVs in their bedrooms have less sex than couples that don't.

As worthwhile as I knew this decluttering would be, it still took me an inordinate amount of time to do it. More generally, this may also apply to you, perhaps with an untidy desk at work, junk in the garage, dirty laundry or dishes in the sink. It can be many things.

Now, I don't believe that we get emotionally attached to dirty laundry or dishes, for instance, where most likely the momentum of procrastination is the main cause. But clutter in a loft, garage or wardrobe does hijack many of us emotionally!

Do you ever have a debate with your good self when deciding whether to give old stuff away, even if you had forgotten it existed and not used it in years? Ever convinced yourself that you should keep it "just in case"? Ever went over the same wardrobe again months later and relived the same debate, yet again? I thought so, and me too.

Why?

Because, to be blunt, we're consumers living in a materialistic society where the things we own end up owning us. Essentially, we're taught that the more we own, the happier we will be. Or perhaps we form emotional attachments to things because they hold some past memories for us.

Either way, throwing out or giving things away is often painful because it represents breaking sentimental bonds to the past or perhaps because we believe we will need them again. It could also point to some belief we hold or even to some insecurity we may or may not be aware of.

Marie Kondo, in her book, *The life changing magic of tidying up*, asserts:

"*Physical clutter adds to our mental and emotional stress*".

Don't believe me?

How did you feel right after the last time you did a spring clean of your home or after you gave away a load of things you didn't need any more to a charity or friend?

Feels good, doesn't it?

That feeling of accomplishment. The re-establishment of some order in your life.

Now, according to self-care coach Eleanor Brownn, *"Clutter is not just physical stuff; it's old ideas, toxic relationships and bad habits. Clutter is anything that does not support your better self"*.

VeryWellMind.com is a useful website that offers some of these tips to eliminate both physical and mental clutter:

- Go through every room in your home and throw away papers, expired food, broken gadgets, etc. Try not to think about it; just do it.

- Donate or sell defunct furniture, shoes or clothes you no longer use. A good rule of thumb is: haven't used it for a year? Give it away. Ouch!

- Avoid buying multiples of things. As enticing as it may be to stock up on sales items, avoid cluttering your home with them.

- Try to spend 10 minutes a day tidying up. Vacuum one room or empty the dishwasher. Doing so saves you from feeling the need to waste a few hours doing it all at the weekend instead, plus it gives you a sense of achievement.

Eliminating Mental clutter:

- Believe it or not, everything described above re. eliminating physical clutter will also help to relieve mental clutter.

- Should you feel overwhelmed by scattered to-do thoughts or random ideas, consider consolidating these into a physical, handwritten list or perhaps into a voice memo recording. This will enable you to better prioritise the more important thoughts or ideas and discard the less useful ones.

Listing will also help to reduce the stress associated with trying to remember too much information, by enabling you to decant thoughts out of your head without the fear of forgetting.

- Take a break from social media; turn off your phone's notifications and limit screen time on your tablets, computers and TVs. This is particularly important first thing in the morning and last thing at night. Please understand, our Homo sapien brains are not designed to handle the vast array of information so readily accessible on our handsets.

- Keep a strong support system of friends and family around you. And if anyone you know exhibits negative energy, cut them out of your life if you can. If you can't, for instance, a family member, minimise contact.

- Create your own 'quiet space' or sanctuary where you can escape your noisy or stressful surroundings or consider factoring into your daily or weekly routine walks in the park or countryside, for instance, to escape the world's distractions.

And finally...

- Adopt healthy lifestyle habits such as daily exercise, drinking plenty of water and a healthy sleep routine. For instance, maybe walk to the train station a couple of times a week instead of taking the bus or make your bed first thing in the morning so that you can start off your day with an achievement, a win.

Declutter your life.

3. BEWARE: Digital Dementia

"Many of us outsource our 'smarts' to our smartphones"

When was the last time you used a physical map to find your way from A to B?

When was the last time you memorised a phone number or a shopping list?

When was the last time you picked up a dictionary?

Chances are a very long time ago. Nowadays, all that kind of stuff is being outsourced to our smartphones.

Now smartphone technology is driving incredible progress. Entry-level smartphones nowadays run rings around the technology that first put a man on the moon.

The problem, however, is partly information overload.

Following on from what I said earlier about reducing mental clutter, memory coach, Jim Kwik, states that using a smartphone is *"like trying to take a sip of water from a fire hose".*

Yes, our brains get a dopamine hit, but they are just not designed to take in all that information. There is too much choice[8] and too much distraction as side-tracking adverts or social media news streams. How the hell can we focus on any one thing?

And the problem is this will also spill over into other non-digital aspects of our lives. No wonder smartphone overuse leads to anxiety.

As well as information overload, your smartphone is replacing both short and long-term memory. We no longer need to memorise directions or numbers or diary dates or appointments. So, our brains are losing their edge. We are losing our mental capacity, and our focus, and society is suffering from what Jim Kwik dubs:

DIGITAL DEMENTIA.

Your brain is like a muscle. Use it or lose your sharpness, your focus, and your attention span.

The more I use my phone, the harder I find it, for instance, to focus on conversations or to take in what I've already read. So, I will often find myself needing to ask others to repeat themselves or to reread the same page of a book two or three times. And I'm much more

---

[8] Anyone else also get stressed by long restaurant menus?

distracted, so I will walk into a room and forget why the hell I went into that room in the first place! Can you relate to this?

Now, if you use your smartphone to free up your brain to do bigger and more important things instead, great. If you just use your smartphone as a memory prop and you don't take opportunities to put your brain to work on the bigger, more important things, you are not exercising your brain, and it will atrophy.

So, what can you do?

Exercise your brain more and rely less on outsourcing your smarts to your smartphone. Keep that brain active to counter the effects of digital dementia.

Here are tips:

- Try to read at least 30 minutes a day.

- Try not to rely on your smartphone too much for undertaking some basic tasks (that won't clutter your mind), for instance, directions when driving to places you will visit more than once.

- Challenge your brain daily with crosswords, puzzles or sudokus to keep it 'plastic'.[9]

---

[9] aka neuroplasticity: the brain's ability to change and adapt.

- Rest your mind by unwinding or partaking in meditation, for instance. Like muscles, resting the brain optimises its peak performance. I'll describe some very basic breathing techniques later on.

And here are three 'digital detox' strategies from author and life coach Jay Shetty:

- Become aware of how much time you spend on your digital devices. Like a diet does with food, know what you are consuming and how long for. Perhaps use a journal to note how much screen time you spend on Instagram or Facebook. Prepare to be in for a shock! Raise your awareness and know that something may need to change.

- Create digital-free zones in your home. Shetty removes tech from his kitchen and bedroom so he can better focus on social interactions in those rooms (oi oi!). For instance, in his kitchen, he can better enjoy his social company and food and "live in the moment".

He even locks his phone outside in his car, so he is less tempted to grab it. Perhaps you can instead start by leaving your phone in another room?

Shetty also recommends digital free time, which he schedules into his diary.

- Like a food diet again, do not completely detox or remove digital devices all at once, as this extreme measure will cause the brain to crave the digitally induced dopamine rush even more. Instead, take baby steps. Cut down on your digital exposure gradually. For instance, cut down on Instagram initially for four weeks, then Facebook for four weeks, and so on. This will likely create a longer-lasting solution.

And I'll add a further personal tip here:

- When using your smartphone, there is so much gumph out there (TikTok videos, Facebook ads, fake-news feeds and so on) - where effectively you are at the mercy of clever addiction programmers - that I would instead suggest choosing and paying for good information apps or source websites. For instance, I find a subscription to The Economist[10] is good for high-quality news.

Disconnect from your device; reconnect with your life.

Beware: Digital dementia.

4. Say "no" more

"It's only by saying "no" that you can concentrate on the things that are really important" - Steve Jobs, entrepreneur, Apple co-founder.

---

[10] A weekly source of fact-checked and balanced (I believe) global news.

Do you find saying "no" to people difficult or challenging?

If so, you are not alone.

Many of us would rather say "yes" to things – even to things we would prefer not to do - simply to avoid the discomfort of saying "no". This is because it's in everyone's interest to get along with others. We are herd animals after all. As part of our hunter-gatherer origins, we had to co-depend on others to survive.

Much like stress or fear, we are hardwired to feel or act in particular ways that may no longer serve us so well in these modern times as they did in more ancient, sabre-toothed tiger times.

Or perhaps we just don't want to hurt other people's feelings.

Or we are worried that our boss will think us inefficient if we don't take on more tasks at work.

Or we genuinely want to help others, even if we don't have the capacity to do so.

There are many reasons we'll be inauthentic when we say "yes" to things that we'd rather not do. The problem is this is not healthy because we are not properly considering our own needs, wants or self-preservation.

This doesn't mean, however, that everyone should be self-serving. It means that, as was best said by psychiatrist Dr Nicole Washington: *"Saying "no" is one of the best forms of self-care that we can engage in".*

Why?

Because saying "no" allows us to:

- Create space in our schedule to rest and recharge.

- Engage in activities that align with our goals or desires.

- Set boundaries with friends, loved ones or colleagues.

Essentially, we can better live a more fulfilling life on our own terms.

So, how will we know when we should say "no" or "yes"?

Well, according to **Psychcentral.com**, ask yourself these questions anytime that you are not sure how to proceed:

- Will saying "yes" prevent me from doing something else that is more important?

- Does this project, opportunity or activity align with my values, beliefs or goals?

- Will saying "yes" make me more tired or likely to burn out?

- Will saying "yes" be good for my mental health?

- When am I more likely to accept a request that I'd much rather decline? And so, how can I change this approach?

Okay, so if it is not in our interest to say "yes", how do we best say "no"?

Here are some effective strategies according to **Inc.com**:

- **Just say it.**

Don't beat about the bush or offer crap excuses, as this may provide persistent others with an opening. Don't delay. Provide a brief explanation if you must (the less said the better) but don't feel compelled.

- **Be assertive and courteous.**

For instance, "I appreciate your asking me for help, but I'm stretched too thin right now."

Or

"Thank you so much for thinking of me, but that's not going to work for me."

- **Set boundaries.**

People sometimes struggle to say "no" because they haven't taken the time to evaluate their relationships nor understand their role within the relationship. When you understand the dynamics and your role, you'll be your true, authentic self. And so, you won't feel as worried about saying "no".

- **Put the question back on the person asking:**

This is particularly useful in a work environment. If your boss, for instance, is asking you to do too many tasks you cannot handle, you might say: "I'm happy to do x, y and z. However, I'll need 3 weeks - rather than 2 - to do a good job. How would you like me to prioritise them?"

This way, you will have created a win-win situation where your boss ultimately gets what they want while you can achieve the desired outcome more comfortably and with less pressure.

- **Put your needs first.**

For if you don't, your productivity will wain and you will become resentful. Let us learn from that billionaire investor genius bloke, Warren Buffett, who said: *"The difference between successful people and very successful people is that ==very successful people say "no" to almost everything".==*

Say "no" more.

* * *

Oh my! That's chapter 1 done already. How was it for you?

As you'll appreciate, these principles are pretty basic and straightforward to implement. But only if you are willing to overcome any procrastination, distraction and/or social awkwardness you may have in order to fulfil your desire to improve the quality of your life.

I am, occasionally, distracted by a pinging WhatsApp message that may prevent me from getting ready for bed; or a work colleague will ask me to take on a non-urgent task that, while making their life easier, will prevent me from getting home in time to spend a nice evening in with the Missus; or – as I draft this book – my bedtime will come and go and then I will go to bed too late, annoyed with myself for compromising the next day.

No one is perfect, not even you or I, and so any step in the right direction, no matter how small, is a victory.

You are only ever one step away from changing your life for the better.

CHAPTER 2

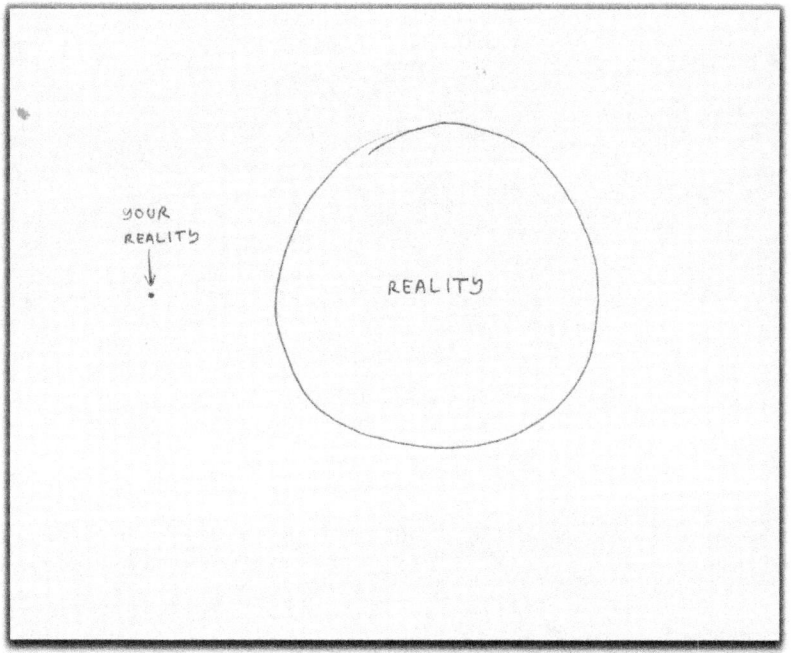

CHAPTER 2
Know thy self

Now that we have established some foundations to improving one's mental and physical health, and before we can begin the outward journeys described from Chapter 4 onwards, we need to ensure that we are as authentic as we can be internally.

What do I mean by this?

I mean, cut the BS.

Discover who it is that you *want* to be. Embrace the things you are most proud of; address the things that need work.

You cannot do any of this stuff, however, unless you are brutally honest with yourself and unless you buck the fuck up. Yes, I just said "fuck", such is the importance of this.

I won't lie; this chapter will likely challenge you big style should you incorporate its principles into your life. If so, you have every chance of coming out the other side a more reliable, better-rounded and thicker-skinned person.

Or maybe you'll instead wind up chucking this book out of the window.

Let's see which it is...

5. Keep your promises

"To be responsible, keep your promises to others. To be successful, keep your promises to yourself" – Marie Forleo, author and entrepreneur.

How often do you make promises to yourself that you'll do something positive in your life?

Perhaps you promise yourself that you'll wake up super early tomorrow morning and go for a jog before breakfast. Or that you'll begin a more balanced, healthy diet in the new year. Or that you'll better manage your time at work so you can spend more time in the evenings with your loved ones.

And how often are these promises, as well-intentioned as they may have originally been, empty and not acted upon?

Or, how often do you make promises to others that deep down you know you have no intention of fulfilling? A deadline at work, perhaps or a pseudo, open-ended coffee date with a friend that was only spoken about because you bumped into them randomly in the street, and it was socially less awkward to feign interest in seeing them again than it was to be authentic.

Well, all of the above has applied to me and then some over the years[11].

I am willing to wager that such streams of broken promises, to both you and others, is something that you will have dabbled in also.

In his groundbreaking book, *The seven habits of highly effective people*, Stephen Covey describes how we each have a circle of concern over which we have little or no control over the things in our life that fall within this circle. But we also have a second circle known as the circle of influence that encapsulates the things in life we do have direct control over. Generally, the circle of influence is smaller than and fits within the larger circle of concern:

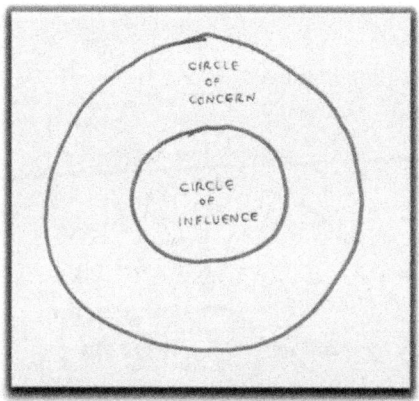

Covey's circles of concern and influence.

In a nutshell, PROACTIVE people focus their efforts in the circle

---

[11] Apologies to any pseudo coffee date friends that may be reading this.

of influence, i.e., they will work on the things they CAN do something about. As they positively develop these things, their circle of influence increases, thus shrinking somewhat the circle of concern:

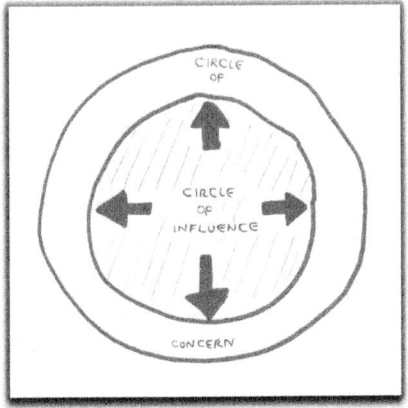

Covey's 'Proactive' circles

REACTIVE people, however, focus their efforts in the circle of concern:

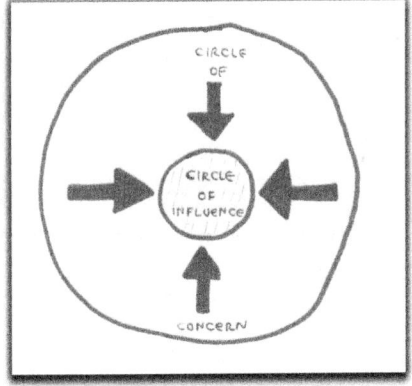

Covey's 'Reactive' circles

Their focus is on circumstances over which they have NO CONTROL. Their focus results in blaming attitudes and increased feelings of victimisation. This NEGATIVE ENERGY causes their circle of influence to shrink.

How does this link to keeping your promises?

By choosing how we respond to circumstances, we may positively affect our circumstances. And, as pointed out by Covey, there are so many ways to work in the circle of influence:

- To be a better listener – and believe me, so few people actually LISTEN! Watch this space as I'll be exploring this later on.

- To be a more loving partner.

- To be a better student.

- We can even choose to be happy.

Yes, happiness is a proactive choice, especially if we accept those things that we cannot control while we focus our efforts on the things we can.

But at the very heart of our circle of influence is our ability to make and keep commitments and promises. The commitments we make to ourselves and others, and our INTEGRITY to those commitments, are the essence of our proactivity. And the essence of our GROWTH.

By making promises and being true to them, we build the strength of character that makes possible every other positive thing in our lives.

Don't believe Covey?

How do you feel deep down inside you when you make a promise to yourself or others that, really, you know you have no intention of honouring? Essentially, you are lying. I suspect, as with me, a little bit of you dies inside because not only have you lost the trust of others, but more significantly, you no longer trust or respect yourself.

To finish in Covey's own words:

As we make and keep commitments, even small commitments, we begin to establish an inner integrity that gives us the awareness of self-control and the courage and strength to accept more of the responsibility for our own lives. By making and keeping promises to ourselves and others, little by little, our honour becomes greater than our moods.

Keep your promises.

Ouch. The truth hurts, doesn't it, unless you strive to be more truthful to yourself and others.

6. Be yourself

"Be yourself, everyone else is already taken" – Oscar Wilde, poet and playwright.

Let's begin this principle with the words of the social psychologist Erich Fromm:

> *Today we come across an individual who behaves like an automaton, who does not know or understand himself, and the only person that he knows is the person that he is supposed to be, whose meaningless chatter has replaced communicative speech, whose synthetic smile has replaced genuine laughter, and whose sense of dull despair has taken the place of genuine pain.*
>
> *Two statements may be said concerning this individual. One is that he suffers from defects of spontaneity and individuality which may seem to be incurable. At the same time, it may be said of him he does not differ essentially from the millions of the rest of us who walk upon this earth.*

Stephen Covey distills this down further:

Essentially most people do not act like themselves – their true selves; instead, they act the way they think that other people think they should act.

This is a mind-blowingly perceptive statement worthy of being re-read a few times.

Many people are, therefore, not authentic.

Mark Manson goes even further in his book, *The subtle art of not giving a fuck*, when he says:

People reconfigure their entire personality depending on the person they're dealing with.

And what is ironic is that you may well not even be right about what other people genuinely think of you.

Generally, if you have low self-esteem or low self-confidence, you will likely assume that others consider you to be weak, untrustworthy, thick or just a plain waste of space. And so, your insecurity or negative self-judgement is based on what you think others think of you, which is a pretty weak foundation.

I'm afraid to tell you that you are not that important. Rather than thinking about you, most people are instead worrying about what you think of them.

A story:

A friend – I won't give her real name here, so let's just call her Annie – went to a Rammstein (a German heavy metal band) concert recently, and she bloody loved it. She called me up straight after the show to tell me how great it was and how happy she was that she pushed herself to stand at the very front of the arena crowd.

Now, if you know anything about Rammstein, believe me, standing at the front requires courage. Anyway, her voice was a-shake with euphoria and adrenaline because she had experienced a positive and life-changing event.

She spent the next few days on 'Cloud 9'... all until something happened.

She had some builders working on her house later on that week and, as she likes to do, Annie was playing her music playlist in the background when Rammstein came on, to which one of the builders told her to turn it off. When she asked him why, the irritated builder went off on one about how he found the language Rammstein used in their songs to be obscene and offensive and that Annie had poor taste in music.[12]

Anyway, without going into detail, he picked on the wrong person because a big argument ensued. Unfortunately, though, what started

---

[12] Please note, I am sanitising what the builder actually said.

out as euphoria had turned into despair. 'Top of the world' had become 'down in the gutters.' All because a person had voiced his subjective, harsh judgement on both Annie and her taste in music.

Annie had allowed someone else to determine her outlook and mood, to hijack her happiness, her self-belief and confidence. This person projected his own concerns and character weaknesses onto Annie; he did not reflect her true character. I tried explaining this to Annie at the time, but it was way too late; the damage had already been done.

The tough lesson here is that you shouldn't allow other people's opinions to influence how you feel.

Strive to be less reactive because, as Covey puts it, reactive people build their emotional lives around the behaviour of others, empowering the weaknesses of other people to control them – as Annie did here.

Proactive people, while still influenced by external stimuli, choose their responses based on their own internal values. These internal values do not need external validation from others. As Eleanor Roosevelt observed:

No one can hurt you without your consent.

And to quote Covey further:

It is our willing permission, our consent to what happens to us, that hurts us far more than what happens to us in the first place. I admit this is very hard to accept emotionally, especially if we have had years and years of explaining our misery in the name of circumstance or someone else's behaviour. But until a person can say deeply and honestly, "I am what I am today because of the choices I made yesterday," that person cannot say, "I choose otherwise."

If you take nothing else from this chapter, hell - this entire book - please take this:

It is not what happens to us, but our response to what happens to us that hurts us.

Powerful stuff, innit?

Ignore what other people think of you and decide for yourself whether you like your own music, whether you're a good parent or partner, whether you're amazing at your job or whether you are socially confident.

If you decide you could improve your performance in your job environment, don't be insecure. Do something about it.

Perhaps you can try out different strategies, ask your peers for help, or if, for example, Excel spreadsheets are an important part of your job, but you just can't get the hang of them, do training courses to address this.

Or, if you can't get passionate about your job full stop, maybe consider changing jobs to something that you do enjoy and hence will more likely thrive in. But don't jump ship until you have first found your shore (new job).

These things, according to Richard Templar's book, *The rules of living well,* will get you to a point where you know you're good at your job so you can then take responsibility for feeling confident and secure about it.

Your proactivity will enable you to no longer rely on anyone else to guide how you feel.

This can apply to social confidence too, where you can learn ploys or strategies that will enable you to stretch your comfort zone. Maybe push yourself to publicly ask that burning question at the end of a seminar, or, instead of hiding behind a WhatsApp message, maybe you can chase up that late electrician with a direct phone call.

In the interests of balance, Templar has one final tip:

If you can't rely on other people's poor opinions of you - real or perceived - you can't rely on their good opinions either.

Compliments, admiration and respect are very nice, so enjoy them but don't ever let it be a substitute for your own honest self-appraisal.

Be yourself.

Yes, yes, I know. All this is much easier said than done, but no one here said that the correct path would be the easiest path. And no one ever made any worthwhile progress without first stretching their comfort zone, which, not surprisingly, is an uncomfortable thing to do.

7. Don't compare yourself to others

"Ever seen a really obese person in a Nike 'Just Do It' T-shirt and chuckled to yourself? Well, don't. You are the equivalent in some other aspect of your life."

I'll never forget a joke that stand-up comic Ardal O'Hanlon[13], once told at one of his shows:

"Did you ever have a friend that won the national lottery, and then you kinda wished that they died?"

This was pretty funny to me and the rest of the audience.

---

[13] The egit priest in Father Ted.

Why?

Because deep down, despite this being an extreme scenario, we could all relate to it. It is human nature to automatically compare ourselves to others, even though we may not necessarily be aware that we are doing it.

We either:

- Look up to people who we consider superior to us in some way, to people who we believe are living a better quality of life than us. A life we can only dream of having one day, perhaps. These will likely be celebrities or friends posting on Facebook or Instagram, showing off their amazing beach holidays, their new cars, their amazing new homes or even their new faces!

Or

- We look down on people who we consider our inferiors, people we believe are living a lower quality of life than us. Perhaps they have less money than us, a crappier car, or they may live in a dodgier part of town. Or maybe they are suffering from ill health or some other hardship we have never known.

And sadly, it is human nature to feel bad or think less of ourselves when we perceive others to be doing better than us. Conversely, we feel better about ourselves when we perceive others to be struggling or doing worse than us. Such an unfortunate human trait, as neither end of this spectrum serves us particularly well.

Shame on you!

While perhaps reflecting on the misfortune of others may offer you a broader sense of perspective and make you appreciate that your lot isn't so bad, ultimately, comparing yourself to others is all about you. About your insecurity, your lack of inner peace or fulfilment. That need for a negative external reference to make you feel good about yourself.

And how much do we know about that person whose lifestyle we envy? Maybe they worked bloody hard to get to where they are today; maybe their amazing job means they never get to spend any time with their loved ones, or perhaps they have a tragic backstory. While you're busy envying the good stuff, the whole picture may be something totally different.

And likewise, the complete opposite may be true of that person you consider your inferior. They may be loving their professional or family life.

We just don't know.

Focusing on what you perceive other people to have will never bring you happiness because, unbeknown to them, you are essentially entering into a competition with that person. And guess what? You will always start behind them. You are unnecessarily putting yourself into a position of negative deficit. You are downgrading your self-worth.

So, what can we do about it?

Well, aside from practising gratitude regularly (see later), there are a few things I'd recommend:

- Firstly, if someone has what you perceive to be all these wonderful things going for them, perhaps you can use these as motivation to achieve some of these things too. If they have a dream job, for instance, perhaps research that field, then investigate signing up to the relevant training courses to get you on track. Or if they have that amazing beach body or 6-pack, maybe start by assessing your diet or by joining that nearby gym.

Be aware of and investigate those things you think will make you a happier, better person, but never compare yourself to others.

- Secondly, Rule 4 of Jordan Peterson's book, *12 Rules for life*, states:

Compare yourself to who you were yesterday; not to someone else today.

Peterson believes that you shouldn't compare yourself to others because they are not you. They do not have your temperament, your troubles, your family or your abilities. They do not have the things that make you, you.

The only person with all those attributes is YOU.

That's why you should only compare yourself to who you were yesterday because that is a game that you can win, unlike a game whereby you compare yourself to others based on your illusions or your perceptions of others.

It is achievable, and it is healthy to try to be a little bit better today than you were yesterday. Maybe you can get up a bit earlier. Maybe you can use social media less. Or perhaps you can exercise or read a little bit more.

BE YOUR OWN BENCHMARK.

Don't compare yourself to others.

Okay, so sod everyone else. Let's work on ourselves a bit more now!

* * *

8. Limit your limiting beliefs

"As high street bookies will have us believe in their commercials that their typical customer is a thirty-something male model with a nice suit and a full set of teeth, as opposed to the more likely sixty-something, alcoholic, paper bag-swigging shipwreck; so, your perception of reality is nothing like reality."

It was in Oxford on the 6th of May 1954 that Roger Bannister ran the first ever recorded sub-four-minute mile.

No one had ever thought such a feat to be possible until that fateful day. For over a hundred years prior, this was the belief. Many believed that the human heart would first explode before a sub-four-minute mile would ever come, but Bannister proved them wrong.

Guess what happened after that, though. Bannister's time was then bettered within only a few months, and then, shortly thereafter, dozens of mid-distance runners ran the mile in less than four minutes.

Why?

Because Bannister broke the entire world's limiting belief[14] and thus opened the floodgates to a new level of athletic achievement.

---

[14] A limiting belief is a state of mind or belief about yourself, others or the world around you that restricts you in some way.

What are your limiting beliefs?

Here are some common examples of limiting beliefs:

- I'm too old to start a new business

- I'm too young to start a new business

- I'm not smart enough to pass that interview

- I don't have enough time to do the things I enjoy

- I don't deserve to be happy

- I don't deserve to be loved

- No one else has ever succeeded in this task before, so how can I?

I could go on all day, but I think you get the picture. And what do these statements ALL have in common?

Assuming one is not trying to defy the laws of science and nature, they are NOT based on FACT. They are based on subjective beliefs that prevent us from pursuing our goals.

Let's cross-examine one of these limiting beliefs:

"I don't have enough time to do the things I enjoy."

For instance, I have friends (try not to look too surprised!) that I haven't seen in ages, and every couple of weeks, we will WhatsApp message each other with statements like *Let's catch up soon, has been too long, blah blah blah* ... but we never do meet up.

Why?

Because we just don't care enough.

However, if one truly cares about something - a task, a relationship or a goal - one will make time for it by re-arranging or discarding other lower-priority tasks. We all have 24 hours in a day. Believe me, you can fit in the things that matter the most to you if you challenge your self-narrative.

These stories we tell ourselves will also usually prevent us from reaching our full potential. And often, they may be subconscious, so we don't even realise we have them.

Why do we have limiting beliefs?

FEAR.

We are hard-wired to protect ourselves from perceived danger, failure or uncertainty. So, we will tend to invest energy into those actions that we believe will produce results. When we don't expect results, though, we often give up before we even begin!

So, where do limiting beliefs come from?

I touched on this in the introduction: past experiences, parents, social circles, schools, media, etc.

Let me give a simple example of how a limiting belief may have been created and then is played out with a tale about a baby elephant in a circus.

This baby elephant is tied to a stake stuck in the ground. As the baby elephant tugs at the rope, it cannot break it or pull the stake out of the ground.

Even though the baby elephant will eventually grow up into a powerful adult that is easily strong enough to just pull out the stake and walk away, it doesn't because it believes that it can never get away.

This is known in psychology as 'learned helplessness'. A limiting belief has been created.

According to MarkManson.net, we also often use our emotions as a basis for our limiting beliefs. For instance:

- *I can't meet new people because I'm too depressed and so no one will like me.*

Or

- *I can't go back to work because I'm too embarrassed.*

But, as Manson observes, there's a paradox within these limiting beliefs:

- *If you're depressed or sad, getting out and socialising may help to destroy your depression or sadness.*

- *If you're easily embarrassed, facing the judgment of others is the only way to get over that embarrassment.*

Ironically, what we need to do to deal with these emotions is the very thing we're avoiding doing.

Again, not based on fact.

How do we overcome our limiting beliefs?

Manson offers these tips:

- Ask yourself: What if I'm wrong?

Limiting beliefs will lose their power if we consider that they may not be true. Can't get a promotion because you're not smart enough? What if you're wrong?

Adopt the ability to question your own beliefs and find alternative possibilities. Challenge yourself to imagine the world where your assumption is incorrect.

- Ask yourself: How is this belief serving me?

Like the elephant from earlier, generally, we hold onto limiting beliefs to protect ourselves from struggle and failure. Victim-mindset people will also hold on to limiting beliefs because it makes them feel special or deserving of special attention:

"It's not fair that I can't change careers because I'm too old - pity me!"

Beliefs should only stick if they serve us in some way. Figure out how your belief is serving you and ask yourself whether it's really worth it.

- Create and test out alternative beliefs

Come up with ways in which you may be wrong. Sure, maybe you're older than most people who start a new career, but who says you can't be successful? It is only your mind stopping you.

Why not try writing down your assumption and then come up with some possible alternatives? For instance, perhaps your being older means you have greater previous working experience to offer your new career? Or perhaps, starting a new business when you are young will offer your business a fresher, new perspective.

This enables you to not only identify your limiting beliefs but also to recognise that you have options.

To quote Manson here:

With repeated practice in noticing your limiting beliefs and imagining new ideas to replace them, you'll start to notice the thousands of tiny little decisions you make based on your limiting beliefs without even realising it. You'll start to notice that the same limiting beliefs that keep you from looking for a new job are the ones that keep you from ordering the sandwich you actually want to eat or wearing the clothes you want to wear - and you'll see how ridiculous it all is. And that's when you'll have more control over what you choose to believe.

And finally...

- Test your alternative beliefs to see if they might be true.

Until we're willing to see if these alternative beliefs play out in the real world, we can't be sure of what is true and what is not. And most of the time we will find we were actually wrong about our initial belief.

As Manson concludes:

It simply takes the self-awareness to consider that we may have been wrong and the courage to go out into the world and see if we were wrong. Challenge your own understanding. Test new ideas. There is ALWAYS room for growth.

Limit your limiting beliefs.

So, what does your less limited self look like?

The world is your oyster, my friend, but only if you're willing to take full responsibility for your own outcomes. Only if you're willing to break up what is seemingly set in stone with a TRUTH HAMMER. No, I've no idea what a 'Truth Hammer' is either, but it just feels right here as the description for the means by which you validate whether your beliefs are serving your greater good or not.

If you found that one pretty tough going, you had better drink a camomile tea and sit in a comfy chair before reading on, as this next one is really gonna boil your bananas!

9. Embrace criticism

"To avoid criticism, say nothing, do nothing, be nothing"- Elbert Hubbard, writer and philosopher.

As I'll describe in greater detail later on in 'Pause, aim, fire', humans are illogical, egotistical creatures that, for the most part, will be unable to receive contrary feedback from others in a manner that is both constructive and free from emotion.

This does not mean, however, that one shouldn't strive to embrace criticism regardless, especially as there are lessons to be learned that may be of benefit.

Just before we get stuck into this, criticism, as negative or harsh as it sounds, can also be used in a positive, constructive way to improve something, not just in a negative way that may lower your self-esteem or cause an undesirable emotion, such as stress or anger.

The shame is most of us on the receiving end of criticism will sway toward the negative response because ego is hardwired into our self-identity.

Kain Ramsay, in his book, *Responsibility rebellion,* has a healthy way of looking at criticism that I am going to describe here because it will help to explain why one should stop taking offence from criticism but instead look to learn from it.

As Ramsay explains, criticism from anyone can be a bitter pill to swallow, whether it's a negative online review of this book, for instance, God forbid, or an opinion from a friend, but not all criticism is ill-intentioned.

Just because your partner offers you some fair criticism every so often doesn't mean they don't love you or want the best for you, and just because your line manager at work gives you some harsh feedback, it doesn't mean that you need to quit your job.

As tempting as it is to label all forms of criticism as hypocrisy, ignorance or spite, Ramsay believes there is ALWAYS some truth to the criticism you receive.

Yoda voice: "A controversial statement, that is!"

O.
M.
G.

While this does not mean that all criticism you receive is accurate, all criticism stems from somewhere rooted in reality. People's accurate or inaccurate criticisms of you are based on their perceptions of you.

So, instead of taking offence, all external criticism should be followed by self-reflection, most especially on how you present yourself to certain people. No matter how crazy, unjustified or wildly inaccurate you may believe the criticism to be, Ramsay believes that discarding it or taking offence is both ignorant and unproductive. Double ouch.

Instead, all feedback you receive is an opportunity to self-reflect and learn about yourself. For you can learn the following three 'Hows' from your critics:

- How you are perceived by others.

- How your behaviours and emotions unintentionally come across.

- How to effectively and ineffectively critique others.

* * *

How can you benefit from criticism or feedback?

By putting your emotions or personal feelings to one side and by being grateful for the insight into an alternative perspective, regardless of how upsetting this feedback may be. And try not to focus on how the criticism was delivered - I mean, there are some pretty emotionally unintelligent people out there. Instead, focus on what you can take away from the criticism without becoming emotionally attached to it.

And, as Ramsay reflects on in another lesson from his book, feedback is a critical stage of the learning process more broadly. This is because true learning cannot take place within a bubble or within a group of like-minded people that do not offer opposition or alternative perspectives. For instance, most of us on Instagram or Twitter will only follow others that share our political or social ideologies, to cement our own beliefs. This essentially means we are shutting ourselves off to growth, to potentially novel, better or healthier concepts or perspectives.

Instead, Ramsay encourages us not to be afraid of listening to all perspectives to learn about them, understand the psychology behind them, and strengthen your own position in accordance with them.

To finish on one of his quotes:

Never block your ears from listening to feedback, even if you'd never believe or agree with it. Your growth and wisdom depend on listening to others, hearing what they have to say, and making your own independent judgment based on the information you have at hand.

Embrace criticism.

10. Be responsible ("response + able")

"Most people do not really want freedom, because freedom involves responsibility, and most people are frightened of responsibility" - Sigmund Freud, founder of psychoanalysis.

You know, I wasn't originally going to include this principle, but after having reviewed the first draft of this book, it was crazy to me how responsibility was such a prominent reoccurrence, yet it didn't have its own principle...so, here's Johnny!

I passed blood in my urine.

It was a couple of months into the first big Covid-19 lockdown and so one can imagine how overwhelmed the medical services (NHS in the UK) already were. So, I called the non-emergency medical helpline, and they rightly advised me to chase this up with my local GP surgery so that they would run tests and take it from there.

I wasn't too worried at the time because I'm very much a "I'll worry when they give me a cancer diagnosis" kinda guy vs. "Oh shit, Google tells me I have two weeks left to live!" But I appreciated that time was of the essence. Anyway, I used my NHS phone app to report my symptoms locally to get a follow-up call.

A week later, nothing. I called the GP surgery and spoke to the receptionist, who assured me that I'd get a follow-up call, but one never came. It took my chasing the GP surgery three further times before they finally arranged for me to have a urine test. Anyway, thankfully, Google was wrong, and I was right.

The reason I bring this up here is that while I have been heavy-handed in this book dishing out some hard truths about how important it is for one to take responsibility for their own outcomes, this example demonstrates the difference between *fault* and *responsibility*.

While it was the NHS's *fault* no one replied to me, it was my *responsibility* to keep chasing them until they fulfilled their function to maintain or treat my health. It was how I responded to their lack of action that ultimately led them to act.

To steal from Spider-Man, and every other wellbeing or self-help podcaster/author out there that seems to use this example, while Uncle Ben told Peter Parker:

"With great power comes great responsibility."

We mere humans should instead consider:

"With responsibility comes great power."

By forcing yourself to force the issue, you have the power to influence the outcome, be it good or bad, even if the circumstances leading to that point were out of your control.

* * *

Now there are some harsh self-help guides and podcasters out there that will tell you:

"Everything is your fault."

And I can relate to this because, as I'll touch on later in 'Pause, aim, fire', between stimulus and response, you have the ability to choose your response. You are responsible for your response.

Response + able, remember?

And, as we dabbled with in 'Embrace criticism', you will never be able to please everyone all of the time because some things you do will just rub them up the wrong way. Full stop.

However, it won't be your fault if a plane crashes into your house or if the person you pissed off is emotionally immature. It is how you subsequently handle the ensuing shizzle that *is* your responsibility, though.

So now that we have established the difference between *fault* and *responsibility* let's focus on the latter, which *is* within our control.

Why is taking responsibility so important?

- Productivity

Things get done when people accept responsibility for their outcomes. My urine test from earlier, for instance.

- Belief and character

Belief in our ability to determine our outcomes is so very important to our wellbeing as well as our emotional and mental health. If we believe that we can change and, where necessary, improve ourselves and/or our situation, we are less bound to our limiting beliefs and so will more positively respond to life's challenges.

This self-development builds character because we will demonstrate to ourselves and others that we don't just talk a good talk. We act. We do.

- Relationships

Taking ownership of our actions, including our mistakes, will improve our relationships with others, which is also key to our better wellbeing and all-around health. For others will consider us more honest, reliable and more worthy of respect.

Why do people avoid taking responsibility?

There are several reasons, some of which are listed below and none of which will surprise you:

- Fear (again)

Some people - that pass blood in their urine or find a lump where it doesn't belong, for instance - would not chase up their medical services for fear of a worse-case-scenario diagnosis.

I'm currently dealing with a building contractor that is trying to charge me for some faulty refurbishment work. Sometimes I think it would be much easier to just pay up and shut up for fear of pissing this guy off or giving myself more hassle by having to micromanage his work.

Or your work colleague may blame you for some shitty work outcome that they're afraid to claim responsibility for.

This is all very easily done, by the way, even when we know that the potential outcome may be far less favourable than taking responsibility, i.e., a long-term health issue or even death, being conned or loss of trust and respect.

- Lack of belief/Low self-esteem

Unless someone believes they can change, they are unlikely to take the first step required to change, which is admitting to and taking responsibility for their mistakes or behaviours.

- Trauma

A traumatic backstory will lead some to adopt victim mindsets (see later), and so their emotional state will trump their desire to take responsibility to determine their own outcomes.

Or perhaps, they were punished for their mistakes in the past, when they were children, for instance, and so admitting their mistakes now is unfathomable to them. Insert fear again here.

- Laziness

Some people are just lazy fucks. They lack motivation and so may not consider whether or how their actions (or lack of) are affecting themselves or anyone else. Much easier to sit back and not help grandma take out the bins or not cook a non-microwaveable meal sometimes. I'm knowingly over-simplifying here, as a 'lazy fuck' diagnosis is likely interspersed with fear and low self-esteem.

There are plenty more reasons we may refuse to accept responsibility (entitlement, perfectionism, etc.), but *War and Peace*, this book is not!

How can we be more responsible?

It would be easy to say you should strive to be the opposite of all the things I've listed above, but that would be both lazy and irresponsible of this author!

- Accountability

Be accountable to yourself. Keep your promises. Admit your mistakes. Honestly, reflect on whether your actions or behaviours are the *right* thing to do or are fairly serving you AND others, regardless of how hard these may be to implement. As the next chapter's introduction will touch on, gossiping behind someone's back is hardly a responsible person's behavior, even when it may be more socially acceptable to your peers.

The next chapter's 'Don't be a victim' principle will discuss how destructive the act of blaming others or complaining is to one's character. If someone else at work gets that promotion over you, learn from it, accept it and move on.

- Commit smartly

Only commit to those things you know you can do, either currently or with further learning, resource or development. By managing expectations, recognising their own limitations, and by knowing when to say "no" (Chapter 1), responsible people will demonstrate to others that they can be relied upon and are trustworthy.

Many will value trust over love.

- How would you feel?

Consider the perspectives of others. What if you were them? What character traits would you look for in someone you were to start a business with, for instance? Then, this is what you should consider others would expect from you.

- Overcome procrastination

Success, in all areas of your life, will rely on your taking the action steps towards that success. You will therefore need to cut procrastination out of your life. Less internet or social media browsing, more reading. Less sitting around doing sweet FA, more walking or exercise. Less lounging around feeling sorry for yourself, more taking the bull by the horns.

- Consistency is key

Chapter 3 begins with a variation on the following theme but for now, let's take it at face value:

How you do anything is how you do everything.

Responsibility is no different.

Strive to be responsible in all areas of your life, not just at your place of work or when you're around your children, for instance. This is because it is a broader sense of personal responsibility that underlies character, and it is your strength of character that will help you to overcome life's challenges.

Be responsible.

How does all this sit with you?

On paper, the 'Know thy self' principles we've just run through may seem paradoxical. First, I'm saying you should ignore what other people think of you but then I'm encouraging you to embrace what others think.

Furthermore, it is easy to believe no one could know you better than you know yourself, and so what can they possibly tell you about yourself that you don't already know?

Answer:

Everything and nothing.

You can take or leave the views of others, but only after accepting that they may have something new to offer you that your subjective self may not see, but also, no one can make you feel any way you do not want to feel.

You and you alone are responsible for your own outcomes.

You should not require external validation, but you should always be open to external perspectives that may expand your horizons or better enable you to strengthen your own position.

Let's pop along to Chapter 3...

Chapter 3

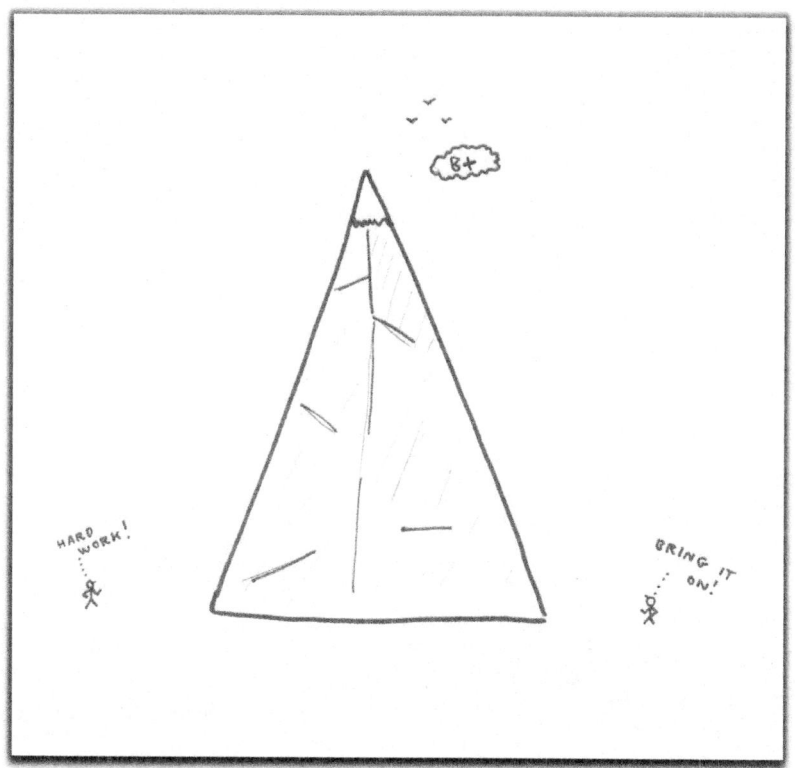

CHAPTER 3....
Are you positive?

How you do anything is how you do everything.

This is a well-known saying.

For this chapter, though, I'd like to adapt it to:

How you see anything is how you see everything.

Let me chuck a little science at you:

Essentially, it's your **RAS**. No, I'm not talking about a night out on the piss. I'm talking about your 'Reticular Activating System' that links the subconscious parts of your brain to the conscious. If, for instance, you buy a red Tesla car, pretty soon you will see red Teslas everywhere because you'll have been 'switched on' to red Teslas. Previously, you may not have noticed them anywhere near as much.

What you focus on expands.

So, if you're a negative person, you will see negativity everywhere. Problems. You won't trust others. If you're a positive person, however, you'll see the good in others, in the small things, in life more generally...so you will likely live a more fulfilled life.

U C WHAT : TAHW U R

* * *

I'm not a spiritual person. I'm not religious. I don't believe in heaven. I don't believe in God. I genuinely wish I did, though, because it would mean I would get to see my dad again one day, and it would take some pressure off of my trying to pack as much as I can into what I believe will be my one and only shot at life. But alas, I believe not so.

However, I strongly believe that whatever one puts out into, for want of a better word, the 'Universe'[15] - be it positivity or negativity – one will get back again but in greater abundance.

This means that positive people will tend to live happier and more fulfilling lives than those miserable fuckers (we all know our fair share of them) that will instead expend their energy by slagging other people off or by blaming everyone or everything else in the world for their woes. And sadly, it's so much easier and more comfortable for most of us to join in with office gossip about absent work colleagues, for instance, than it is to either defend these absentees or just not get involved.

Doing the wrong thing (joining in) will always be the wrong thing, though, and doing the right thing (defending or ignoring) will always

---

[15] Yes, I know, 'Universe' sounds way too airy fairy for my liking also!

be the right thing.

So, bringing this back to the general positive or negative stance, you have the following choice:

a) I choose to be a positive person grateful for the blessing that is my life; that sees the good in things; that will always strive to offer patience and empathy.

or

b) I choose to be a negative person, cynical of the world and suspicious of others; everything that is wrong with my life is outside of my control; my problems are the fault of others.

Okay, so these choices are at the extreme ends of the spectrum as many of us fall within 'the grey' but most of us would agree that we would prefer to hang around with people that fall within the A group.[16]

The principles of this chapter will describe how to move yourself away from 'the grey' or even the 'B team' (miserable fucker) to the upper echelons of the lightest shade of grey where you'll be knocking on the driver's door of the A-Team van.

---

[16] As long as their positivity is general; not delusional!

Just before you recover from that well-placed A-Team reference, let me add the caveat now that this chapter is NOT endorsing 'toxic positivity'[17] nor is it for one second saying that adversity or negative experiences don't often lead to personal growth, because they do (chapter 6); it is instead saying that a healthy mindset and outlook is everything.

Right, let's get this plan together!

11. Shift your perspective

"When you shift your perspective, suddenly the life you're living changes" - Mandi Briggs, Simplymandi.com.

I once got a speeding ticket and, in order to not get any penalty points on my driving license, I had to attend a speed awareness training course run by the police (in the UK, this is). At one stage, the police trainer asked my group what driving situations we found ourselves in that made us drive in a more irritable or dangerous manner. And then, he asked us to think about how we could best address these issues.

My key example was being late for an appointment and then being stuck behind a really slow driver or perhaps a driver late to move away from the traffic lights. Other than managing my time better in future, one solution I came up with to address my impatience was to

---

[17] An unrealistic, extreme form of positivity that is NOT healthy.

SHIFT MY PERSPECTIVE the next time I was stuck behind a slow driver.

What if the person in front of me had just lost a loved one?

What if they had just come back from a cancer diagnosis?

What if they were frail or elderly?

Or

What if they were depressed and having a bad day?

I have since found it interesting how a simple shift in perspective alone has helped to bring out my better, more patient side.

* * *

In his book that I've mentioned, *The seven habits of highly effective people*, Stephen Covey describes what he calls one such paradigm[18] shift he experienced: One day, he was sat on a New York subway train. Everything was peaceful and civilised, and then, suddenly, a guy got on with a couple of children. The children proceeded to run amok in the carriage, screaming and grabbing at people's newspapers, causing a crappy change in what was previously a

---

[18] The word 'paradigm' is from the Greek for "frame of reference".

pleasant atmosphere. The man seemingly oblivious to all this, just sat down next to Covey with his eyes closed. Covey felt himself getting more and more irritated as the children continued to tear up the carriage while their insensitive father just sat there doing nothing. Eventually, Covey snapped and turned around to the guy and said:

"Your children are really disturbing a lot of people, can you not control them?"

To which the man lifted his gaze for the first time and softly said:

"Oh, you're right. I guess I should do something about it. We just came from the hospital, where their mother died about an hour ago. I don't know what to think, and I guess they don't know how to handle it either."

Imagine being in Covey's position.

He had an abrupt change of perspective or a significant paradigm shift. Suddenly he saw things differently and so he thought differently, felt and behaved differently. Essentially his irritation vanished and was immediately replaced by both compassion and sympathy. Everything changed in an instant.

Now many people experience a similar fundamental shift in thinking when faced with a life-threatening crisis or when they step into a new role, for instance, a first-time parent.

The lesson here is that the map - aka your perception - is not the territory because it is impossible for you, me or anyone to have the full picture or to know the full story of everything happening around us.

So, the next time someone winds you up or irritates you, please take a moment to consider what may be happening to them in their lives; something that may not be at all obvious to you. For to do so, will help to unlock in you a humanity and compassion that may otherwise have lain dormant.

* * *

I will add another angle here which crosses over with the 'Limit your limiting beliefs' principle of chapter 2 and that is beautifully encapsulated by the following John Archibald Wheeler quote:

As our island of knowledge grows, so does the shore of our ignorance.

True depth of knowledge essentially will be reflected by an appreciation of just how little we know in the grand scheme of things, including alternative perspectives.

Beware that person that believes they are at the top of their game; that they know all they need to know, and so person will close themselves off to challenge, feedback or new ideas. Beware. For this is how ideologies are formed.

As we touched on in the previous chapter's 'Embrace criticism' principle, expand your horizons by looking outside of your peer group. By following people on social media, for instance, which may have different beliefs or persuasions to you, you will be better placed to challenge your own limiting beliefs or knowledge.

And whenever entering into a challenging negotiation or discussion, prepare for it by first considering what the other person's viewpoint may be. As convinced as you may be of your own position, what possible harm could it do to challenge this position from as many alternative perspectives as you can think of? No matter how crazy or unlikely these perspectives may seem at first, give it a go. Who knows, you may change your mind or, at the very least, better be able to get your own point across.

This is a powerful skill you can develop through practice. You can even have some fun along the way too. Why not get together with some friends and play a game where you write down some unlikely statements that you will need to either argue for or against? The winner being whoever can come up with the most compelling arguments. For instance:

- Pavements or sidewalks should be made of jelly;

Or

- People should be readily allowed to sell their bodily organs to whoever wants to buy them.

Two extreme statements, perhaps, but challenge yourself to argue in favour of them. I bet you'll surprise yourself with what you can come up with!

***

Let's wrap up this principle with one final thought experiment:

Can you imagine a situation where one could have feasibly sympathised with a Nazi soldier? Unlikely I'd say, and with good reason, too, given the scale of atrocity inflicted by the Nazis on the modern world.

Well, my dad was about 8 years old when his village in Italy was occupied by the Nazis during the final years of the Second World War, and his family had to survive day-to-day. Food was scarce, crops were uncertain, and people were being executed. These were unimaginably frightening times for my dad. Yet when I asked him about these, it was his unexpectedly fond recollections that stood out for me. For he told me of times when young German soldiers (in their teens and there against their will), when ordered to leave the village to head to the front lines, often had to be dragged away kicking and screaming from the older Italian villagers who had taken these boys into their homes and who had loved them as their own. Villagers who had sometimes even lost their own sons to the war.

Such a rare incite I include here because it demonstrates a glimmer of humanity, via an unexpected perspective, in an otherwise overwhelmingly dark history.

Nothing is completely black or white.

Shift your perspective.

The world could do with a little more compassion and patience in it, so why not give this principle a whirl? You'll likely find that it'll bring with it some inner peace when you push yourself to look at the behaviour of others in a more balanced, empathic way. Or maybe you'll learn something new and unexpected along the way that will improve your life.

* * *

12. Watch your self-talk

"Be very careful what you say to yourself because someone very important is listening. You" - John Assaraf, author.

This one is based on personal observations.

How many times have you made what you perceive to be a stupid mistake, and then you beat yourself up about it afterwards?

You've probably called yourself an idiot (or likely much worse) after spilling coffee over your lap or perhaps after saying something that you then regretted. Perhaps you'll also physically reinforce this by shaking your head to yourself. Worse still, you may then have a crappy day or, if we will go all out, you then make the lives of others around you crappier too!

Here's an example:

I play football or soccer a couple of times a week, and I have lost count of the number of times I have seen other players make a mistake, for instance, they miss a penalty, and then they spend the rest of the game on a downer: they play worse; they are more volatile; they are shouty; they are irritable and, most annoyingly, their negativity puts a massive drain on the rest of their team's performance.

Negativity is contagious.

Perhaps you work in an office where the dynamic would otherwise be great were it not for that one negative colleague that literally spoils it for everyone else because they bring out the negativity in others too. Misery loves company.

Watch your negative self-talk and physical signalling and try to catch yourself before it slips out and impacts on you and those around you.

I'm still working on this bad boy myself. For instance, I recently left my phone in the car and cursed myself for having to go back out of the house and into the street again to retrieve it. Not a big deal in the grand scheme of things.

One strategy I've adopted since then, though, that works for me, is: I either catch myself mid-negative outburst or immediately afterwards, and I cancel it out by doing the exact same thing again but from a position of positivity. So, if I say: "FFS, what a bloody loser leaving the phone in the car!" I will immediately respond with something like: "So what, big deal, I'm a caring and generous person!" This response, if applied with genuine self-respect, can serve to not only neutralise the negative deficit but it may also switch you up a gear into a more positive mood. And say it out loud so you can hear the glowing self-affirmation. Granted, you may get funny looks if you're out and about, but who gives a toss what other people think when your happiness or positive mindset is at stake?

And, as per numerous self-help books out there, frame your thoughts in positive words and language.

For instance, "And" instead of "But": "I went to the supermarket, *but* I forgot to buy the bread" detracts from the fact that you may well have brought loads of other things you needed. However: "I went to the supermarket, *and* I forgot to buy the bread" is framed better. By using "And" you make it more likely that you will also come up with a solution, i.e., there's more to come, whereas "But" is more final and negative.

There are loads of other such word reframing examples: try swapping "Should" to "Could" as *could* gives you more control of the situation vs *should* which implies someone else is making you do it.

And please steer your self-talk away from final outcome words such as "Always" or "Never ever" because this implies that you are without choice, flexibility or options. How many times have you said: "That's just like me to *always* forget the bread"? Well, a) this is probably not true and b) oh shut up!

Watch your language and self-talk.

And whilst I'm on the subject, a controversial one, I'm afraid: Don't make a habit of apologising to others unless you have genuinely wronged them in a significant way that requires you to take full responsibility for yourself, and unless you genuinely mean it. While this humility and self-deprecation is a very British thing that seems deeply embedded into our culture, it is nonetheless a sign of weakness as it also puts you in a negative deficit. For you are telling others, and more importantly, yourself, that you have done a noteworthy wrong and so may be untrustworthy, time and time again.

And have you ever noticed how we Brits, when asked how we're doing will often respond with: "Not bad, thanks" whilst our American counterparts will often frame their responses more positively with: "I'm good" or "I'm great"? But anyway, I'll leave it there for now.

- Catch your negative self-talk before it consumes you and others.

- Practice your positive self-talk to put yourself in a healthier, happier and more productive mindset.

And

- Don't apologise unless you have acted like a proper shit and unless you mean it, as to do so makes you come across as a weak people pleaser, and so you may lose the respect of others.

Watch your self-talk.

This next principle has a financial wealth component to it but I'm hoping you'll appreciate the parallels with mindset wealth.

13. Don't be a victim

"People will throw stones and hide their hands and then get back and play victim" - August Alsina, singer.

T. Harv Eker's book, *Secrets of the millionaire mind*, is the most powerful book I have ever read regarding financial wealth mindset. And one of the main reasons for this is that his wealth principles have a much broader application than money wealth alone.

Briefly, this book is a no-nonsense, easy-to-follow guide on how one should steer clear of the poor person's **SCARCITY** mindset to achieve the rich person's **ABUNDANCE** mindset.

Caveat alert:

'Poor' or 'Rich' as in **MENTALITY**; not the amount of money we have or our value to society. It just so happens that a poor mindset, more often than not, precedes financial weakness, whereas a rich mindset precedes financial success.

* * *

In one of his, what he calls 'Wealth files', Eker observes that rich people believe "I create my life" whilst poor people believe "life happens to me."

Eker says that if you want to create financial wealth, it is imperative you take full responsibility for your financial life. Unfortunately, the poor mindset person chooses to play the role of the VICTIM instead. And victimhood leaves 3 clues:

- BLAME

Victims blame the economy, the government, the stock market, they blame their manager, they blame their employees, they blame their partner, their spouse, they blame Covid, they blame God, and they blame their parents. It's always someone or something else's fault, never theirs.

- JUSTIFICATION

The victim may justify or rationalise their lack of money by saying such things as: "money is the root of all evil" or "money is not really important." As Eker rightly points out, if you tell your husband or your wife they are not important to you, would they hang around? No. And neither would money. And, although love may make the world go round, it doesn't pay for building homes, hospitals or churches. It also feeds nobody.

And finally

- COMPLAINING

Eker believes that complaining is the absolute worst possible thing you could do for your health or wealth.

Why?

Because what you focus on expands. By complaining, you are therefore focusing on and expanding all that is wrong in your life. As I said at the start of this chapter like attracts like, negative attracts negative, crap attracts crap!

Keep away from complainers!

And if you're a complainer yourself, you will find general success hard to come by, so you will need to work hard at **NOT BEING A COMPLAINER**.

Please indulge this author by doing one of T. Harv Eker's homework assignments he believes will change your life: For the next seven days, you will strive to not complain. Not just out loud, but in your head as well. And for seven full days.

Why?

Because you will be amazed at how much better your life will be when you stop focusing on, and therefore stop attracting, crap into your life.

And now for my own addition: If someone has done you a wrong, addressing that to their face takes character, and it takes integrity; bitching behind their backs does not. Tough, but you know I'm right!

To close with some wise words from Eker:

From now on, as you blame, justify or complain, try to cease and desist immediately. Remind yourself that you are creating your life.

Don't be a victim.

Just when you thought I was already putting too many demands on your integrity and positivity, I've only gone and titled the remaining two principles of this chapter: 'Practice gratitude' and 'Focus on the positive.'

14. Practice gratitude

"Let us rise up and be thankful, for if we didn't learn a lot today, at least we learned a little, and if we didn't learn a little, at least we didn't get sick, and if we got sick, at least we didn't die; so, let us all be thankful" – Gautama Buddha, founder of Buddhism.

What are you grateful for today?

If your answer to this question is "nothing", please find a quiet place where you won't be disturbed, sit the fuck down and slowly read aloud this principle. Such is its importance to your quality of life:

Gratitude is different things to different people.

Gary Vee, entrepreneur and podcaster, for instance, wakes up every morning and checks his phone. If none of his top 10 most important people in the world have died, he is so grateful that he cannot help but have a good day from that point onwards because his gratitude eclipses other less important stresses.

Or, as a friend, Nico, once reflected on, many of us will say things like:

"I *have* to go to work."

Or

"I *have* to go to the gym."

When instead we ought to reframe by saying:

"I *get* to go to work."

Or

"I *get* to go to the gym."

While tying in with 'Watch your self-talk' from earlier, such statement variations will matter less to someone fully mobile and more to someone confined to a wheelchair, for instance.

And so, it transpires that most of us will take all manners of things for granted UNTIL these things are endangered or taken away from us. Imagine your clothes, shoes, chairs, the roof of your home, your water, food, bed, sofa, electricity, etc., all disappearing right NOW. Would you then no longer take them for granted?

YES.

Do you know how many people are involved in the process of getting clean drinking water running to your taps or how many people it takes to plant, grow, bake, package, transport, stock and then sell your favourite potato crisps or chips to you? Like me, probably not, but I'm guessing lots of people.

People in 'poorer' third world countries will more likely not take ANY of these things for granted, which goes some way to explaining why, on average, they are likely to live more purposeful lives than the rest of us 'fortunate' ones.

And what if you knew that you would only ever spend one final weekend with your parent, partner or child, for instance. How much more grateful would you be for that weekend?

I'm thinking much more grateful, as every small thing about that weekend would become much more significant. Your Instagram feed or bank balance would likely become far less important to you.

And so, as we'll touch on again in the final chapter, given that our time is finite and that most of us have no idea how much time we have left, surely it would make the most sense not to take any weekend, day or moment with our loved ones for granted.

Lack of gratitude explains why most of us will instead spend much of the next weekend with our loved ones gawping at our fucking phones, scrolling through social media bollocks that will add absolutely nothing positive to our lives.

* * *

Yet have you ever noticed how good news – such as a positive outcome to a stressful situation, for example, a successful job interview or an overturned cancer diagnosis – will put an extra spring in someone's step? Suddenly everything else doesn't seem so bad by comparison, such is the power of gratitude.

Can you guess where I'm taking this?

If we can carry this gratitude around with us at all times, we can live happier, healthier, more fulfilled lives.

Jim Kwik says:

If a person could do only one simple thing to increase their health and happiness, then expressing gratitude regularly must be it.

Perhaps then we should practice gratitude daily.

Today, for instance, at the time of writing this, so far, I am grateful for the nice coffee and breakfast I shared with my Missus, the good morning message my mum sent me on Facebook messenger, the sunshine outside that made my cycle to work more pleasant, the lunch break I shared with my work colleagues and the wonderful and unexpected catch-up phone call from my mate, Joe, that made my day. Plus, I am grateful that I can create this book for you, dear reader.

So, when me and the Missus go to bed at night (oi oi), we will each take out our journals and spend 5 minutes or so writing down 10 things we are grateful for from that day. When writing my top 10 gratitude list, each item goes something like:

"I am so very grateful for X (whatever the thing is) because Y (the reason you are grateful). Thank you."

For instance:

"I am so very grateful for the "best ever coffee" compliment from the customer that came into my café today because it made me feel valued. Thank you."

Maybe you can do this too by gratefully reflecting on your day at the end of each day.

You don't need to journal if you don't want to, as even spending a just few moments thinking about these things you are grateful for is great too, though journaling has its advantages:

- Writing down your thought forces you to spend longer thinking about it.

- You need to think about it properly to write down the reason you are grateful.

- You can read it back to yourself again afterwards so you are doubly grateful.

- You will likely get more restful sleep and perhaps even a better start to the next day because of closing your day with some positive thoughts.

And

- If you ever have a low moment where you feel like the world is against you, you can throw open your notebook and remind yourself why you are blessed.

Please note that earth-shatteringly impressive things don't need to happen in your day for you to fill your gratitude journal. Perhaps you can be grateful for your good health that day or for a nice shower you had.

* * *

And if I may throw in a curve ball, aside from outright tragedy (although one may argue otherwise), one should also strive to find gratitude within more difficult circumstances.

Why?

Because, as unfathomable as this may seem at first, there is wisdom to be learned and opportunity to be gained from challenge. For instance, if your romantic relationship breaks down, perhaps you can be grateful for all the times when the relationship was good; perhaps you will now have some much-needed time for self-reflection, or, if you lose your job, perhaps you can be grateful for all the experience you have gained from that job or for all the other jobs out there.

Taking this up a notch, Kazimierz Dabrowski, a Polish psychologist that studied how Second World War survivors handled their post-traumatic experiences, noted that many believed themselves to live happier and more fulfilled lives afterwards because the horrors of the war taught them the power of gratitude and the non-importance of life's trivialities. Trivialities that many of us today will allow to rule our lives.

I'd start with practising the good stuff first, though, as perhaps only a seasoned practitioner of gratitude would be able to appreciate the magnitude of the previous paragraph!

Remember what I said earlier in this chapter about like attracting like, be it negative attracting negative (crap) or positive attracting positive (fluffy stuff)? The same goes for gratitude. Greater gratitude brings with it greater inner peace and fulfilment.

Then, the key to greater inner peace is applying this gratitude across as many aspects of your life as you can.

Please try not to take anything for granted. Especially this book ;)

Practice gratitude.

15. Focus on the positive

"Only in the darkness can you see the stars" - Martin Luther King, Jr., civil rights activist, minister.

Simon Sinek, author and speaker, once spoke about a time when he and a friend were attending some busy event where the event organisers were handing out free bagels to the crowd. There were long queues where lots of people wanted to get their free bagels. Sinek grabbed his friend and said that they should get in line, also. When his friend realised how long the waiting time was, he said that they should leave instead, to which Sinek said:

"But I want my free bagel."

His friend replied:

"Yeah, but the long queue."

To which Sinek said:

"Free bagel, free bagel!"

Essentially, whilst Sinek's mate could only see the inconvenient queue, Sinek could only see the prize that awaited them should they be patient enough.

The point Sinek assigned to this story was that their perspectives were different. They were both looking at the same thing; they merely had different views. It's like two people climbing the same mountain; one sees the hard work ahead of them, whilst the other one sees the prize that awaits: the summit. One is focussing on the *how*, whilst the other is focussing on the *why*. As per the next chapter's 'Find your Why', your *why* should come before your *what* or your *how*.

And those people that primarily focus on their *why* are the more positive and proactive people amongst us. They are not deluded, nor are they ignorant of the challenges that lie ahead of them; they just realise that the prize beyond their challenges justifies their challenges.

And be honest with yourself: Would you rather surround yourself with positive or negative people? "Positive people" should be your answer because they bring out the best in you too. They bring out your more positive attributes. You should cut negative people out of your life or at least try to minimise contact.

And, of course, this means you should strive to be the positive person in other people's lives, also.

* * *

Author and psychologist Kain Ramsay, whose work I mentioned earlier, describes in one of his life coaching courses some core skills he employs when he counsels people. One skill is being 'positive outcome focused'. This is because many people will focus on the negative, on the past. It is imperative that a counsellor or coach is positive outcome focused by looking forward and asking questions that get people to STOP looking at the things they DON'T want but instead START focusing on the things they DO want.

For instance, one powerful counselling strategy that Ramsay describes is to listen out for when someone describes negative things that have happened to them in the past. Negative things they will dwell on and allow themselves to be defined by. He will then respond by asking them whether there are any lessons that they can learn from in the past that they can then build into their future. And he says it's amazing how many people are blown away by this, as they will literally *shift perspective* in front of him.

Sadly though, being positive outcome-focused goes against how much of society will often think. Office gossip, for instance, is rarely positive and paraphrasing what Ramsay says, this is why the news is only geared towards negative things. Because this is what society thrives on.

Try not to watch the news if you can help it, and most especially not if you suffer from anxiety or a low mood.

But anyway, the role of a coach or counsellor is to shift people's focus away from all the doom and gloom by being positive outcome focused. This is a simple, yet fundamental tool anyone can use to help others.

So why is positive thinking so important?

According to VeryWellMind.com, it can have a beneficial impact on both physical and mental wellbeing. Those of us that have a more positive life outlook will more generally cope better with stress, have improved immunity, and have a longer life expectancy. And a positive mindset will promote greater feelings of happiness and fulfilment.

* * *

Let us defend humanity a little bit here!

Fear is hardwired into all of us because it's a survival tool remnant, left over from when we were hunter-gatherers. The problem is, outside of more extreme life-death scenarios, this ancient instinct is less necessary nowadays, but it persists nonetheless and so will create our needless stresses, anxieties and inevitable mental health issues.

So how do we work on developing a more positive outlook or mindset?

- Practising gratitude is a powerful tool here. As per the previous principle, don't forget to recap regularly all the things you should be grateful for every day.

- As per the 'Watch your self-talk' principle, studies by Kross et al[19] have shown that positive self-talk will positively affect emotion and will better equip you to handle stress.

And finally

- As the motivational speaker Jim Rohn once famously said:

"Stand guard at the door of your mind."

This means you should pay attention to the thoughts that you have each day.

And should your thoughts be negative?

Strive to replace or reframe them with more positive thoughts. For instance, rainy weather brings my mood down sometimes, so I'll reframe it: Today was so hot and humid, the rain has cooled everything down again so I'll sleep better tonight, or I don't need to water my plants today, or the sound of rain can be relaxing to listen to when I'm in bed.

---

[19] Ethan Kross et al. J Pers Soc Psychol. 2014 Feb; 106(2):304-24.doi: 10.1037/a0035173 (zzzzzzzz)

And please try to remember the following important fact:

Thoughts are just thoughts.

Sometimes, we just can't control what pops into our heads. This is normal. Everyone has bad or negative thoughts, some days more than others. We all have negative thoughts we wouldn't dare share with others for fear they would be shocked or that they would harshly judge us.

BUT we can choose whether to validate these negative thoughts or not. Whether we wish to feel guilty or not. Whether these thoughts serve us or not.

And if they don't serve us, we can learn to replace or reframe them.

Stand guard at the door of your mind.

***

In the interests of balance, and as I touched on at the start of this chapter, positive thinking can have its occasional downsides also. Being unable to accept any negative emotions, aka 'toxic positivity', can have a detrimental effect on both yours and the mental wellbeing of those around you. For, by inflicting toxic positivity on others, they may find their feelings dismissed or invalidated.

So, while it's important to have a positive outlook, look to manage your expectations by being realistic in your approach. Don't set the bar too high, too soon. Instead, raise it incrementally.

Focus on the positive.

Is it just me, or we did we breeze through this chapter a little too quickly?

Perhaps this is because you abound in positivity, and so this chapter merely serves as a refresher!

If not, that's okay too, as hopefully, you will appreciate the broad mental and physical health benefits that come with trying to be a more patient, optimistic, grateful and, generally, a more positive person.

This won't always be easy, though.

'Negativity bias' is the well-known notion that even when of equal emotional intensity, negative occurrences will have a greater impact on one's psychological state than positive emotions. This isn't helped by there being a far richer, more descriptive vocabulary surrounding negative experiences than there is for positive experiences.

Furthermore, it can be difficult sometimes shifting your perspective, focusing on the positive or feeling gratitude when things aren't going so well in your life. For instance, we've all been at the receiving end of a tongue-lashing from a stressed person, or how can one ever expect to be optimistic following a terminal cancer diagnosis?

Albeit completely differing circumstances, these are both understandable predicaments. Though I would ask:

What benefit does negativity bring to either situation?

None. Alienation from a work colleague or partner, perhaps, or a more miserable journey for you and your loved ones under already very difficult circumstances.

And what benefit would positivity bring to either situation?

Potentially lots. You would be more respected and loved for not taking out your stresses on others, and you would likely overcome your stresses more quickly and effectively. And you would be better able to make the most of the valuable time you have remaining with your friends, loved ones and yourself.

In recent years I have lost relatives to terminal illness, and the ones that will always stand out for me are the ones that faced their lot head-on, with integrity, peace and acceptance. And without fail, these were always the ones that lived their healthy lives authentically and as positively as they could.

* * *

CHAPTER 4

CHAPTER 4
What actually matters?

I want you to think about what it is that actually matters to you.

Have you recently thought about what your purpose is?

Are you enjoying your job?

Are you enjoying your life?

Are you doing everything you can to live your best life?

If not, why not?

These principles will equip you with some simple tools that will better enable you to blow the "If not, why not?" question out of the water and replace it with a new question of your own:

How can I address all of these things?

* * *

16. Live with the end in mind

"Believe in the person you want to become" - *unknown.*

Please take a moment to picture yourself at the funeral of the person you love most in this world.

Picture yourself getting out of the car dressed in your formal funeral attire, and you walk into the church, chapel, temple, crematorium, whatever. As you walk to the front of the hall, you pass everyone that you consider significant in your life: your friends, uncles, aunties, cousins, and work colleagues, and as you get closer to the front, you see your mourning parents, siblings, partner or spouse.

Try to imagine the stinging pain of deep sorrow in the room and the warm glow of shared love for the deceased.

You then head to the open casket sitting on the altar and you look inside:

You see yourself.

Please take a moment to picture all of this. Closing your eyes may help.

And then, take another moment to reflect on what you would like the eulogy to say about you. The collective eulogy of all the people of significance in your life. What would you want them to say about:

- Your character.

- Your contribution to their lives.

And

- Your achievements?

I recommend you take a few moments to draw up a list on some paper or on your phone's notes.

Please put this book down or pause the audio for a few moments while you do this.

* * *

Back in the room!

Would you like to know what's on my collective eulogy list?

- Under character, I said: kind, generous, loving, thoughtful, positive, witty, creative.

- Under contribution: lit up people's lives, helped others, love, music, books, podcasts and a loving husband, sibling, son, friend.

- Under achievements: being a good person that made a positive difference in people's lives.

And what struck me most about this simple exercise was that it reframed my definition of what I previously considered personal success.

I didn't mention money, qualifications, recognition, fame or any of the material things that most would associate with success. Instead, I mentioned the things I consider deeply important, which for the most part, entailed positively affecting the lives of others.

Interestingly perhaps, when I ran my eulogy list by a friend, she told me it sounded like I was putting too much emphasis on pleasing others and not enough emphasis on pleasing myself. To which I replied something along the lines of I'm not there yet, but I believe that when someone is truly comfortable and at peace with themselves and their lives, they don't dwell on what others think of them and, invariably, a by-product of inner peace is that others will automatically think more highly of them. For instance, if in future this book becomes successful - and by 'if' I really mean 'when' - then a by-product of my efforts will have been the positive contribution to the lives of others. Perhaps even you, dear reader.

So now I say this: If you know what is deeply important to you, why don't you do everything within your power now, today, tomorrow, to make it happen? To make it a reality?

According to Stephen Covey:

So many of us get so caught up in the activity trap - the busyness of life, working so hard to climb the ladder of success - that we may only realise much later on that the ladder was leaning up against the wrong wall.

PLEASE DON'T BE ONE OF THOSE PEOPLE.

When you live with the end in mind, you gain a different perspective. If you carefully consider what you wanted to be said of you in the funeral experience, you will find your definition of success.

Well, what are you waiting for?

Take some steps in the right direction!

Live with the end in mind.

Okay, so you should've just spent a few moments on this exercise and received some sort of prod in the general direction of personal fulfilment. If not, chop chop. I'll be here waiting for you.

→ here (me waiting) ←

Now let's get a bit more specific.

17. Find your why

"He who has a 'why' to live for can bear almost any 'how'" - Friedrich Nietzsche, philosopher and philologist.

What is it that gets you out of bed in the mornings?

What is it that drives you to do your 9 to 5 job, day in, day out, for most of your waking life?

Or let me ask you again:

What is your purpose?

What is it that fulfils you the most?

What is your 'Why'?

Would you be surprised if I told you that most people I ask either:

- Just don't know.

- Never really thought much about it.

- Have some preconceived response, such as "I want to make loads of money" or "I want to get married and have kids."

Or

- They give me several answers as a stream of consciousness, where they seem to be figuring it out in front of me.

This is all crazy because surely your purpose in life - your Why - should be a pretty fundamental priority for you!

And, before we move on, saying stuff like your purpose is to make money or have kids rarely brings the fulfilment that comes with discovering your personal sense of purpose. True purpose is not a specific end goal. It is more of an ongoing impact on the world, small or large. Journey, not destination.

It is your purpose - your Why - that sustains you through thick and thin. Purpose gives you stability and direction which is why finding your Why is essential for living a fulfilled and healthy life.

Ideally, your purpose blends with what interests you and brings you joy. In Japan, this concept is known as IKIGAI and essentially entails finding the overlap between WHAT you LOVE, and the WORLD NEEDS with WHAT you are good at and the WORLD will PAY for.

If you're lucky (or driven), you find your Ikigai through your job. For example, a paramedic may believe their purpose in life is to help the sick or suffering. Others, however, may get caught between work, family and social expectations, and so they abandon what they consider the unrealistic, idealistic version of themselves.

Finding your Why in life is not just a 'nice to have' though; it will contribute to your better all-round health.

Figure out a way to clearly articulate to yourself what your Why is, as to do so will more quickly put you on that road to fulfilment! Or, to reframe it, knowing your Why enables you to filter out all the unnecessary crap or distractions in your life so that you live with greater clarity and inevitably greater energy that will better see you through rainy days!

* * *

Simon Sinek's book, *Start with Why*, and his many excellent TED talks, describe what Sinek calls his 'Golden Circle', which he says is a simple formula used by all successful leaders and organisations:

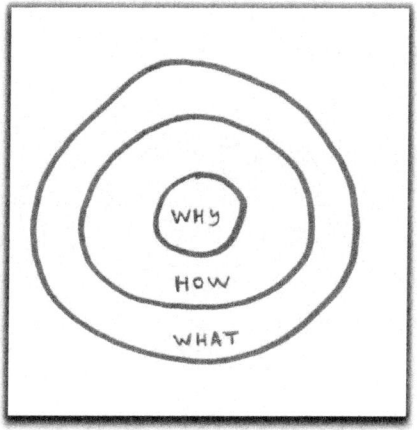

Sinek's 'Golden Circle'

The smallest inner circle or core is your <u>Why</u>, aka your purpose/your motives; the slightly larger middle circle is your <u>How</u>, aka your methods; and the largest outer circle is your <u>What</u>, aka your results or outcomes.

Sinek says that your Why should come first when communicating, before your How and your What. For instance, a company such as Apple is massively successful because it puts its Why first. Its Why being innovation and thinking outside of the box. All this before it builds its computers, iPhones, iPads, or before it counts its profits.

The mistake that most other companies or leaders make, however, is that they do things the other way around. They start with the What, aka profits, then they move on to the How i.e. they build their computers or products, and they may then not even think about their Why! And this is their big problem because people or consumers care a hell of a lot more about your Why or your motives than they do about your What or your How.

This may also apply to job interviews where your motivational fit, or your motives for wanting the job, should be more important to your prospective employer than your technical skills. Why? Because, unlike technical skills, you cannot teach someone their Why or their motives for doing a great job.

And most importantly, starting with your Why will clear your path to a more fulfilling and successful life.

* * *

Let's put this principle to bed with some tips on how to find your Why:

- Take time to create a personal vision statement, which essentially describes your values, your strengths, and your life goals. This should be reviewed regularly and will give you a sense of inner control over what is happening in your life. This can help you to move from a cycle of stress to one of balance.

- Giving back, or being prosocial, can help develop your sense of meaning and purpose because when you help others, you also help yourself. Look for ways to be of service. Perhaps by volunteering or donating your skills to a worthwhile cause.

- Practice gratitude (yes, yet again) as this can make you more generous to others which ties into giving back as described.

- And finally, explore your passions and interests as these are often a good indicator of the area in which your purpose, your Why, will lie. And, according to Sinek, if you're not sure what your passions are, ask the people who know you best. For it is likely that you're already pursuing these passions without even realising it. And who knows, your passions may become a hobby, a side hustle or even a full-time source of income.

So, take some time to dig deep, my friend, and figure out what it is that you give to the world!

Find your Why.

* * *

18. Look at the bigger picture

"*In the big picture, it doesn't really matter if we never made a record, or we never sang a song. That isn't important*" - George Harrison, The Beatles.

So, I went to a new bar near my home recently with the Missus. We'd separately walked past it a few times before but agreed that, given how convenient it was with regards to where we live, we would explore it together in the hope of discovering a cool new, local hangout.

As we walked in, we noticed that their happy hour - 2 cocktails for the price of 1 - finished at 7 pm. It was 7 pm at that moment, so, perhaps cheekily, you may say, I asked the waiter whether they would still honour the happy hour deal if I ordered our drinks immediately. Embarrassingly for us, he made a big show of looking at this watch, then exclaiming that, because it had just gone 7 o'clock, and that his business was a small, new one, they couldn't afford to stretch out their '2 for 1' offer beyond the advertised time. When I politely responded with something like: "Ah, it's only just gone 7. Can't you just stretch it on this one occasion?" His body language switched to 'disgruntled mode' and he begrudgingly replied with something like: "I guess, if you must insist, but the rest will be full price!" He then threw two cocktail menus on to the table in front of us and stormed off.

The Missus and I looked at each other half awkwardly, then we sat down. As we perused our drinks choices, both of us were becoming increasingly uncomfortable at the prospect of hanging around an unwelcoming bar being served by a moody waiter. We were sat there for about 10 minutes waiting for him to return and take our drinks order, but he never did. So, half relieved, we got up, left and then spent an unholy small fortune on cocktails in another bar instead.

The moral of this story for me is that, rather than his investing in our potential continued custom by being nice to us and stretching out his happy hour by one minute, all he could think about was the short-term loss of profit associated with the one cocktail.

Had things gone differently, perhaps we would have become his new regulars that would have told all our friends about this cool new bar. And then they might've told all their friends and so on. He may have subsequently generated significant profits had he handled this one situation differently. He should have responded proactively with an eye on the bigger picture and because it simply would have been a nice thing to do. Not reactively as he did, by instead focusing on the perceived loss.

You know what, maybe, as per the 'Shift your perspective' principle, he just had a really crappy day which we just so happened to crossover with. So, I hold no ill feelings for this individual. However, once burnt, I rarely visit the same bar or restaurant twice if I can help it[20].

The point I'm making - as per 'Pause, aim, fire' (Chapter 5) - is that we should always seek to create a gap between stimulus and response so we may better choose appropriate actions that are more likely to yield longer-term benefits; not a shorter term, fleeting relief.

---

[20] By the way, the bar, should you also wish to avoid it, is called...just kidding, I'd never do that!

If someone spits in your face and you act on an impulse to slap or punch them back, sure, for a split second afterwards, you may feel a bit better. Like you may have somehow recovered your pride (whatever that is), but maybe later on, they'll press charges against you for assault, or maybe they fall back and crack their head open on the pavement (which isn't made of jelly), or maybe this person had a mental health issue they could not control, or maybe things escalate for the worse, and they subsequently kick your ass!

Or how many people, for instance, will immediately sell shares when the markets plummet only to see those shares go back up again and surpass their original value in the medium to long term. They will neglect to look at the bigger picture, the actual reason they invested in stocks and shares in the first place.

Impulsive or short-term thinking, which doesn't involve immediate self-preservation, for instance, jumping out of the way of a speeding car, may well not serve us longer-term.

So, the next time something challenging or unexpected happens to you, try to create enough of a gap between stimulus and response that will enable you to choose the most appropriate course of action that will best serve your longer-term needs!

Look at the bigger picture.

* * *

So that's Chapter 4.

The benefits of considering and then investing in our longer-term outcomes are clear to see. Whether we use the funeral self-reflection exercise to identify some life goals or whether we consider the reactive waiter story, understand that we always have the power, *now*, to lay down whatever foundations for the future we want.

And hopefully, you'll consider identifying your Ikigai if you haven't already done so. Maybe you'll even think about whether what you're doing now is contributing to your purpose, your Why. If it isn't, it may be worth reassessing your current job, situation or activities.

I'm not for one second suggesting, for instance, that you be reckless by dumping your unfulfilling job if this alone enables you to pay for life's necessities. I'm suggesting that you use your free time to research that dream job or lifestyle. That you update your CV or resume. That you take night or weekend classes to give yourself the best chance of getting the appropriate training or qualifications that will land you that interview. Then once you get that dream job, or once that side hustle overtakes your day job salary, only then do you cut free and transition over from all that doesn't serve your ambitions.

This is your one and only shot.

Please make every moment count as if it were your last because you just don't know when that last moment will come.

By not taking anything for granted and by identifying and chasing your Why, only then will you be giving your best to everything that you do.

* * *

CHAPTER 5

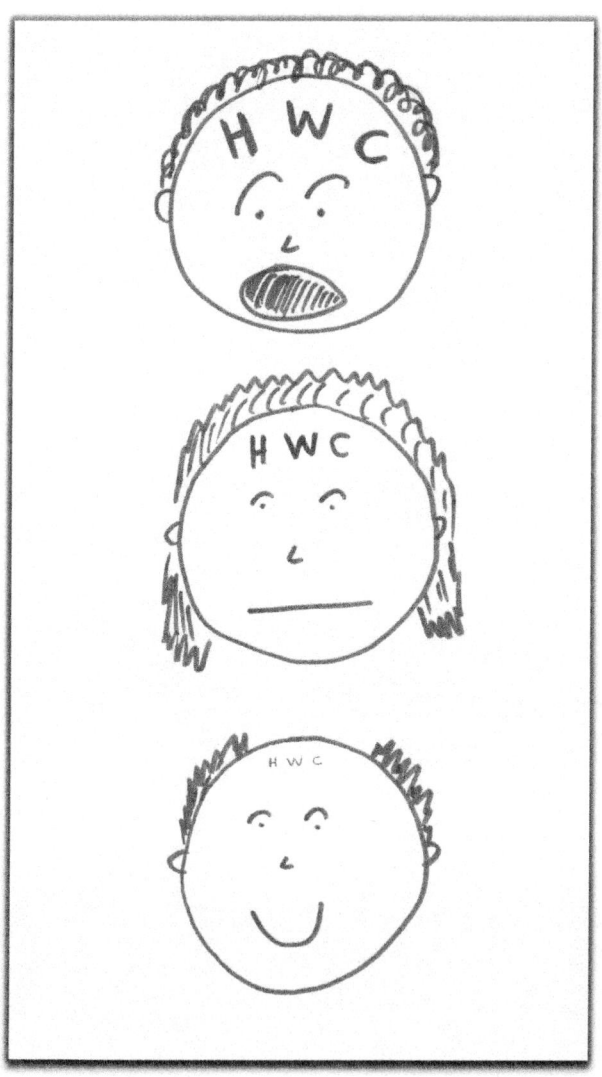

CHAPTER 5

Connection, connection, connection

Okay, we have focused on ourselves long enough. Let us reach out a little further.

Get comfy, as this is a hefty chapter.

This is because social interactions are a major contributor to personal wellbeing, and so I have explored several key areas I feel are important to pin down and understand.

We, humans, are funny creatures, however, that would benefit from tattoos on our foreheads saying:

"Handle With Care"

Some of us would need larger tattoos than others!

* * *

19. Be genuinely appreciative of others

"Appreciation is a wonderful thing: It makes what is excellent in others belong to us as well" - Voltaire, writer and philosopher.

Dale Carnegie's book, *How to win friends and influence people*, is essentially a practical guide to unleashing one's potential to turn around relationships and improve dealings with the people in our lives.

Now, given I am quoting from Carnegie and various others regarding interactions with other human beings, I will add the following caveat: Cynically, one may see these 'skills' or 'insights' as a form of manipulation to get other people to do what you want. While I understand this, as per the last chapters, please try to see these insights from a position of integrity and authenticity. For we are social animals, and so it is in **ALL** our interests and nature to get along with others and mutually flourish. True fulfilment comes from positively and genuinely interacting with others.

But anyway, enough of that! Let's get back to the principle of 'Be genuinely appreciative of others.'

In chapter 2 of his book, Carnegie explains how the human desire for a feeling of importance is one of the chief distinguishing differences between mankind and the rest of the animal kingdom. Freud once said everything you and I do springs from two motives: the sex urge and the desire to be great.

Some of Carnegie's own examples of famous people struggling for a feeling of importance include George Washington, who wanted to be called 'His mightiness the President of the United States.' Columbus pleaded for the title 'Admiral of the ocean and viceroy of India.' And Catherine the great refused to open the letters not addressed to 'Her Imperial Majesty.'

Hell, one reason I'm writing this book is the need to feel important. Deep down, I'd bet even Mother Teresa craved it. We all do!

Where was Carnegie going with this?

If people are so hungry for a feeling of importance, imagine what miracle you and I can achieve by giving people honest appreciation. And I mean honest appreciation, not insincere flattery, which not only will be obvious, but it may well lead to more harm than good.

Now, Charles Schwab, one of America's original steel magnates and one of the most successful business leaders of all time, was asked by Carnegie what his big secret was, and he said:

"*I consider my ability to arouse enthusiasm among my people the greatest asset I possess, and the way to develop the best that is in a person is by appreciation and encouragement...*"

"*... in my wide association in life, meeting with many of great people in various parts of the world, I have yet to find a person, however* *great or exalted his station, who did not do better work and put forth greater effort under a spirit of approval than he would ever do under a spirit of criticism!"*

* * *

When we are not ruminating over some problem or issue, we will spend the vast majority of our time thinking about ourselves. Yes, we are also selfish creatures!

Now, imagine if, instead, we strive to think less about ourselves and more about other people's good points. Then we wouldn't need to resort to false flattery, and we would positively address what, according to Carnegie, is one of the most neglected virtues of our daily existence:

APPRECIATION

A story:

I love a good macchiato coffee avec one sugar. Thank you very much. Unfortunately, go to any chain café such as Starbucks or Costa and their macchiatos (in my humble opinion) will taste more like dishwater than coffee. This is likely because larger franchise coffee houses generally won't put the same time or effort into making your coffee as, let's say, an independent coffee shop would, the latter only thriving if it can make coffee that's good enough to attract repeat, local customers.

'Café Barcelona' is one such local coffee shop near where I live. I'll never forget this one time I went in there for a takeaway macchiato and the barista put so much care into making my coffee: She steam-heated the coffee cup, washed out the milk jug and refreshed it with fresh milk, which she steamed; she then washed out the coffee portafilter[21], topped it up with freshly ground coffee and then ran not-too-hot water through it and into the cup; then she added the sugar, stirred it in; and then carefully finished it by adding the freshly frothed milk. As I walked out of the café, I took a quick sip of my macchiato, and it was one of the best coffees I had ever had. I was genuinely taken aback by this. I turned around and told the barista as much, and you should have seen how her face lit up, such was her beaming smile. She was so grateful that I acknowledged her efforts.

And the next time I visited Café Barcelona, the barista recognised me, was at great pains to welcome me back, and then she made me another amazing macchiato! Win-win!

In Carnegie's own words:

"The next time you enjoy a nice meal in a restaurant, send a word to the chef that it was excellent and when a tired salesperson shows you an unusual courtesy, mention it."

---

[21] Or, as it's technically known, 'that metal handle thingamajig'

"Try leaving friendly trails of little sparks of gratitude on your daily trips. You will be surprised how they will set small flames of friendship that will be rose beacons on your next visit."

And funnily enough, as we sat down to dinner together the other evening, my Missus got annoyed with me because I had forgotten to do some home admin. Without missing a beat, though, as I tucked into my delicious dinner, I automatically exclaimed what an amazing meal she had cooked. I was genuinely gob smacked. It was so good. And, you know what? My chuffed wife so completely changed mood it was unbelievable. At the risk of revealing my big secret, I even mentioned her mood change to her there and then, but she didn't care. She was just so happy that I had recognised her talent and efforts.

* * *

To summarise:

Be genuinely appreciative of others. For not only will people cherish and treasure your words in a way that will inevitably improve your interactions with them, but you may spark a wider and wholly positive chain reaction in their interactions with others.

"Trade your expectations for appreciation, and your whole world changes in an instant." - Tony Robbins, author and life coach.

Be genuinely appreciative of others.

* * *

Isn't it amazing how even the simplest genuine acknowledgement of another's efforts is such an effective means of building bridges with that other person that will improve the lives of both sides?

This shouldn't be too hard to implement if you can deploy in your interactions with others the positivity and authenticity developed in Chapter 3.

Okay, that was easy peasy. Let's take it up a notch!

20. Pause, Aim, Fire

"Between stimulus and response there is space. In that space is our power to choose our response. In our response lies our growth and our freedom" - *Viktor Frankl, psychiatrist.*

How many times have you reacted to a negative emotion in a way that, shortly thereafter and in the cold light of day, you then regretted?

Personally, I've lost count of the number of times I have sent reactive emails to people that have subsequently burned bridges (yes, more bridges). Even after sometimes just a few hours, once the anger, frustration or irritation has dissipated, I look in my sent items box and recoil in horror at what, only a few hours before, I had deemed a completely reasonable and justified message. Too late, the bomb has landed. The damage has been done!

And it's not just emails. I've been in arguments where I have criticised somebody, then immediately regretted it afterwards. But again, too late. Bombs. Damage.

As famously coined by our buddy, Dale Carnegie:

Any fool can criticise, condemn and complain, and most fools do!

So, what should we do when we find ourselves pissed off with others?

We should PAUSE.

Put that harsh unsent email into the drafts folder, hold back from posting that corrosive letter and bite that emotional tongue before the fires of fury are unleashed.

Two simple reasons you should pause:

- Your mind is much less reasonable in its agitated state than it is in its calmer, more rational state. And thus, you are less likely to consider the consequences of your outburst.

- The inevitable resentment that criticism invokes in your friends, family, work colleagues or business associates still doesn't address the underlying cause. Instead, it alienates you. And, assuming your bridges remain intact, you can well expect several roadblocks ahead.

Remember, we humans are not logical creatures. We are instead creatures of emotion, of pride, of ego.

Don't get me wrong. Constructive feedback, when packaged appropriately, can sometimes land successfully to achieve the desired, improved outcome. You'll remember the 'Embrace criticism' principle from Chapter 2, for instance. But be warned: There are some emotionally unintelligent people out there (that may not have read this book), and so even the best-intentioned feedback will sometimes be misconstrued.

Have you ever, for instance, sat in an office with someone that, as part of a management training course, had received anonymous 360° feedback from their peers? I have, and I can tell you: It ain't pretty! For more often than not, most improvements suggested genuinely by peers are not received in the same spirit they were intended. Instead, egos get bashed, personalities become defensive and often, the self-identified victim seeks to identify their anonymous Judases! Ain't pretty...

So, to come around full circle, if measured, constructive feedback can do that to a seemingly rational human being, God help you if you send that email, post that letter or blurt out those words!

Solution:

Pause and come back a few hours or days later to that draft email or letter and reassess it through a more compassionate set of eyes. It is likely that either would need significant re-drafting. Or gratefully reflect on how your self-control held your tongue back during that hot moment.

* * *

Let me briefly share the story here of Viktor Frankl, a Jewish psychiatrist imprisoned in a Nazi death camp during the Second World War. Aside from his sister, Frankl's entire family perished in the camps, and he himself was subjected to horrendous acts of torture. Despite unimaginably difficult circumstances, through incredible self-discipline, Frankl was able to mentally detach himself from his physical situation and look on at his plight as more of an observer than as a victim. He found meaning and dignity in his suffering and was able to develop a now well-known principle based on self-awareness:

Between stimulus and response, one has the freedom to choose.

The Nazis could not take from him what he coined "the last of the human freedoms." He was able to objectively decide for himself how he would respond to his circumstances.

Frankl subsequently taught this 'freedom to choose' principle to others, both during his imprisonment and afterwards.

While I hope that no one reading this book will ever come close to enduring anything like what Frankl did, I hope that the extremeness of his situation will help you appreciate the freedom of choice you have that falls within the *pause* of 'Pause, aim, fire.'

To finish in Dale Carnegie's wise words:

Instead of condemning people, let's try to understand them. Let's try to figure out why they do what they do. That's a lot more profitable and intriguing than criticism: and it breeds sympathy, tolerance and kindness:

To know all is to forgive all.

Pause, aim, fire.

* * *

So, we don't want to hurt people's feelings if we can help it. Instead, we should strive to be less reactive and more considerate of how others may receive us.

Let us now consider a simple principle that will have these very same people eating out of our hands. Not really, but they will like us much more, and so our social interactions with them will improve greatly.

* * *

21. Remember names

"Most people won't hear names because they care more about being interesting than interested."

When I was studying at UCL, I used to regularly meet up with a friend for coffee who I'd been mates with for a couple of years. For some strange reason, though, I never knew his name. Rather than my asking him his name early on, or checking with someone else that would know, I just let it slide...until one day we were just chatting, and I don't remember what I said, but he just looked back at me, bemused, and said:

"You don't know my name, do you?"

I was so embarrassed. I had offended him because I may as well have told him:

"I don't care what your name is because you're not that important to me!"

Do not underestimate how someone's name is to that person, the sweetest and most important sound in the entire universe! Otherwise, why is it that public libraries, art galleries or museums owe their most impressive collections to rich donors who cannot bear the prospect of their names being forgotten after they themselves have long gone? Yes, the average person is far more interested in their own name than all the other names on earth put together.

However, many of us are too busy or distracted, or we simply cannot be bothered to make the time or effort to remember someone's name unless there is a direct benefit to us in doing so. Sad and selfish, really. Shame on you!

Yet history tells us that many successful business leaders, politicians or presidents have attributed a portion of their success to simply remembering other people's names to gain goodwill by making others feel important.

Remember that name and say it to that person easily, and you pay the most subtle yet highly effective compliment. Forget it, misspell it, or worse still, say the wrong name, and you will be at a serious disadvantage!

People rarely care about how much you know; they care about how much you care.

So, whether it's for business etiquette, international networking or social networking, remembering names is an important skill to have.

Jim Kwik, in his podcast Kwik Brain, describes seven quick tips to effectively remembering people's names. He recommends that before heading out to a social gathering or networking engagement, look in the mirror and say to yourself:

"I'm going to BE SUAVE"

- The B in 'Be suave' stands for 'Believe.'

All skills or habits are belief-driven, so never think you're too old or that you'll never be able to get good at remembering names. Believe you can because you can!

- The first E in 'bE suave' stands for 'Exercise.'

While physical exercise feeds your brain, exercise here refers to practice remembering names. Perhaps, you have a list of speaker names at a conference you can try to commit to memory.

- The S stands for 'Say it.'

When you meet someone for the first time and they tell you their name, say it back to them, "Oh, hi, Deborah," so you hear it twice.

- The U stands for 'Use.'

Use the name in conversation three or four times in context. More than that, they'll think you're a psycho!

A stands for 'Ask.'

Most people love talking about themselves so if they have an interesting or unusual name, ask them about it: "Where's it from?" "How do you spell it?"

- The V stands for 'Visualise.'

Our brains are much better at remembering faces than they are at remembering names. So, try to see or visualise the name. If someone's name is Mark, for instance, imagine they have a big bright mark on their forehead or if their name is Mike, imagine them jumping up on a table and singing karaoke into a microphone.

The crazier the visualisation, the more likely you are to remember someone's name.

- And finally, the second E in 'be suavE' stands for 'End.'

Always end the conversation using that person's name "Nice meeting you, Chris."

Remember names.

* * *

If you have any doubts as to how important the names principle is, ask yourself how it would make you feel bumping into someone you met before - who you felt you connected with - yet they didn't remember your name vs. someone who you didn't recall ever having met, yet they remembered your name?

Answers:

Sucks (receiving end) vs. embarrassing (you twat).

My name, Romano (hi), is fairly distinctive in the UK where I live. Yet 9 times out of 10, people I will have met for the second time will get it wrong. An interior designer last week called me 'Riccardo'. Still, I've been called worse!

But on the rare occasions that people will get my name right, I will feel instantly flattered, as they will have considered me worthy enough to be memorable. And so, I will warm to that person much more quickly.

* * *

This next principle is a more serious inadequacy in the human condition yet is so powerfully fundamental to all social interactions.

22. Learn to listen

"I like to listen. I have learned a great deal from listening carefully. Most people never listen" - Ernest Hemingway, novelist and journalist.

As the boring round table meeting at work ran on, the meeting chair turned to me and asked for my thoughts on a particular matter, to which I replied:

"I have nothing further to add to what's already been said."

He awkwardly looked around the table, then came back to me and whispered:

"But no one else has said anything yet."

* * *

Listening is one of those few skills that everyone thinks they have, yet the vast majority of people will never possess.

And to clarify from the outset, hearing and listening are not the same thing. Hearing is the physiological act of hearing sounds - in through your ears and not so much brain work. Hearing is a passive, physical act that does not require concentration.

Listening, however, according to physician and Psychology Today author Kristen Fuller, MD, revolves around actively paying attention to the words and sounds that you hear to absorb their meaning and develop an emotional response. Listening can be defined as hearing something with thoughtful attention. Listening is a voluntary act. If you choose to listen, then it is an active process.

To summarise, hearing is passive, whereas listening is an active process you choose to undertake.

So, even though schools don't teach it (which is bonkers!), what does active listening require? Curiosity, motivation, purpose and effort.

The active listener attempts to internalise and understand what they are hearing to connect with the other person and have a meaningful conversation. Active listening is a prerequisite to understanding and solving a problem with another individual.

Not surprisingly, then, is active listening also a prerequisite to healthy relationships among peers, coworkers, romantic partners, family and friends.

On the opposite end of the spectrum is passive listening, which is characterised by being disconnected, inattentive and unreceptive. A passive listener has no desire to contribute effectively to a conversation. They have likely already formed an opinion, so they are unwilling to work with others to forge a solution. Passive listening is not a good way to communicate with people you are striving to form relationships with. Hence, marriages break down, friendships will be insincere, and inevitably, our mental health will suffer.

Why?

When we choose not to listen to others, we may create a rift in our relationship with that person, be it our spouse, child, coworker, peer or friend.

Perhaps we choose not to listen to someone because we are just too busy, too distracted, or we do not want to hear what they have to say.

Essentially, we are minimising them by telling them that what they are saying, or feeling, is not important to us. By passively listening, we are causing strain on that relationship which can eventually affect our mental health and maybe even that of the person we are not listening to.

But by choosing to actively listen and engage with others, we show them they matter and that we are willing to form an alliance with them. We may see these benefits:

- We can resolve conflicts and create better solutions for the future;

- We can create strong and genuine relationships;

And

- We can understand, exchange knowledge and expand our otherwise limited horizons.

No bloody wonder then that active listening is the cornerstone to any healthy marriage, business alliance or friendship. Active listening is essential to improving your interpersonal relationships.

Can I let you into a little secret?

Sometimes, I am a bad listener because once I think of something to say in response to someone, or once I get a good idea that I think will blow that person's mind, I will try to hold onto that thought or idea so I may tell them about it when they have finished talking. This comes at the cost of actively listening to that person. This isn't good and is (yet another) personal work in progress.

Here's some top tips for you and me to becoming better active listeners:

- Focus

Focus on the conversation by blocking out other thoughts and sounds from your mind to pay attention to the words being spoken. Staying present in the conversation is often challenging, so you will need to limit other distractions. Try putting your phone away, and don't be one of those inconsiderate tossers that instead put their phone face down on the table! Out of sight, out of mind.

- Respect

Have you ever been in the middle of saying something that you thought the other person was engaged with, and then, suddenly, the other person gets distracted by something on the TV or a stranger walking by? I remember once when my dad was ill, for instance, someone asked me how he was, and as I answered them, they broke eye contact and instead looked at someone else walking past with a dog. I must confess it takes a lot to piss me off, but I found that to be particularly disrespectful.

Unless your trousers are on fire, God help your future relationship with that person if you undermine their efforts to engage or enlighten you.

- Ask good questions

Active listening requires asking open-ended questions and genuinely being curious about the conversation. Respond with an "okay", a "hmmm" or an "oh" and it may come across as you're not listening or interested in the conversation. Instead, when someone tries to share something with you, take it upon yourself to learn more by asking thoughtful questions. By asking who/what/where/when/how questions, you are demonstrating that you are listening and that you want to learn more.

And if you find the conversation to be boring, challenge yourself to make the best of it. For sometimes, something completely left-field and unexpected may come crashing out of it that may be gripping and enlightening.

- Wait to speak:

Another thing I do sometimes, that really pisses my wife off, is I will try to finish other people's sentences for them when I feel they are struggling to articulate a particular thought or when I think I know what they will say. Even though people like Gary Vee make a good living from this, I do not recommend it!

Most people in conversation are simply waiting for their turn to speak! We just love the sound of our own voices, and so we often interrupt others before they have finished speaking.

In my own defence, Your Honour, my family is Italian, so a conversation involving five people will often involve five people all talking at the same time!

However, to be a good active listener, we must wait until the other person is done talking and sharing their ideas. There are cues that will tell you when someone is done speaking. Perhaps as visual non-verbal cues or listening to them closing a sentence or a thought. Not only should you concentrate on the words being spoken, but you should also be aware of how the words are spoken. And then you should pause before you share your own opinions.

And finally

- Eye contact and posture:

Eye contact is an important part of face-to-face conversation, as is posture. Try to keep your posture open, as crossed arms, for instance, may make you look closed or defensive, whereas leaning slightly forward, or a slight tilt of your head, demonstrates active listening.

Improve your active listening skills to improve your communication skills and better your interpersonal relationships.

Learn to listen.

* * *

How did that one sit with you?

Did you identify any areas needing work?

If you genuinely didn't, you're likely an emotionally intelligent, well-rounded, and thoughtful individual. I salute you.

If, like me, however, you identified some homework here, give it your best shot. For most people just won't appreciate how critically important a skill active listening is, and that it needs to be developed and then maintained.

God speed.

* * *

Moving on, I learnt this next one the hard way.

23. Don't preach

"Taste your words before you spit them out" - unknown.

There are times to teach, and there are times not to teach.

There is never, however, a good time to preach.

To clarify, and before we get stuck in, Google "Preacher" and it'll spit out something like:

"...a person who delivers sermons on religious topics to an assembly of people..."

However, in this principle, when I refer to 'preaching' or 'preachers', I am referring to people whose message is not about religion but instead about some sort of worldview, be it philosophical or about personal development, for instance. To add my own further spin on it, someone who preaches is essentially someone that tries to impose their own agenda or worldview onto others from, what they perceive to be, a position of superiority. A position of "been there, done that", or "I know better than you, so do as I say!"

And I must confess, the reason I created this particular principle was so you could take something useful away from my own experiences. At the risk of getting myself into some hot water, should they ever read this (they won't), my two siblings have self-destructive tendencies. For instance: they'll have poor sleep regimes (sometimes bed, sometimes sofa in front of the TV) where they won't see morning daylight hours at weekends, or they'll get 3 hours of sleep on weekdays, they do zero exercise, they have poor diets; they never read; etc., etc.!

Now, because I know these things they do, or don't do, are detrimental to their physical and mental health, I have for years, and until recently, been trying to get them to see the error of their ways.

And how have I done this?

I'm ashamed to say by nagging or preaching.

And does it work?

Does it fuck. Course not!

And, yes, in the context of this principle, 'nag' or 'preach' are interchangeable. But anyway, why doesn't nagging or preaching work?

- For a start, it creates resentment.

Because your siblings or your spouse or your child resent you, the last thing they'll want to do is the thing that you're nagging them about. Essentially, they'll be motivated to punish you by not doing it.

I was cycling in the park once (even though it was a 'No cycle' zone - yes, I'm that edgy), and even though the path was about 15 feet wide, a miserable fucker walking the other way and on the opposite side to me, went out of his way to cut across to my side of the path and then shout at me to dismount because I had nearly hit him.

Do you think I dismounted?

No. He had pissed me off and deserved to be ignored as far as I was concerned.

- You will make that person feel controlled or manipulated into doing something against their will. Hence, they will dig their heels in.

- It is exhausting for the recipient because it wears them down, so they'll most likely just shut off or hang up that phone.

- It focuses on what the person is not doing. It has negative focus because it points out all the things wrong with that person. It makes them feel unworthy for not doing certain tasks, which ironically may further contribute to that person's poor mental health. Instead of building them up, you are pulling them down!

- As per this book's foreword, nagging is essentially a more aggressive form of advice-giving, which itself is not healthy.

And finally

- When you preach or nag someone, according to my siblings, it makes you out to be a complete and condescending knobhead.

So, what should we do instead?

- I genuinely believe that some people, sometimes, need to discover the truth for themselves, even if this means hitting rock bottom. And all we can do is love and support them both along the way and afterwards too.

- Make a fuss about and positively encourage the good things that they do do[22], no matter how small, as even small improvements are better than no improvements. And who knows, several small improvements later, and the momentum may carry them forward into bigger, life-changing improvements.

- Once you have distanced yourself from being an established nagger

---

[22] "…do do…" - grammar checker just went ape shit!

(or aggressive advice-giver), you may instead develop a relationship with the other person in which you can prompt them every so often with the odd (subtle) nudge that may get them to re-think things. For instance:

"I don't know how you do it. If I only got 3 hours sleep every night, I'd be a right zombie at work!"

And finally

- Rather than preaching or nagging someone regarding the knowledge or lessons you have learned, *live the message*. Lead by example (without rubbing their noses in it), as people are more receptive to seeing than they are to hearing. Walk the walk and let them see the positive effects in your own life and, who knows, they may follow the same path.

Much like many of the other principles in this book, patience and empathy are very much the order of the day when it comes to dealing with loved ones you feel are letting themselves and others down.

By playing the longer game, you'll see your efforts pay off more effectively, and you will then enjoy seeing your loved ones flourish thus enabling you to flourish with them.

Don't preach.

Okay, let's not avoid the 'L' word any longer!

24. Love is a verb

"You are what you do, not what you say you'll do" - Carl Jung, founder of analytical psychology.

On her way out of the house, my wife tripped up over my bike that was badly parked at the bottom of the stairs. She yelled as she fell over, so I immediately rushed downstairs to see what all the fuss was about. Fortunately, she didn't break anything (herself, my bike), though she was bruised and shaken up. She was properly pissed off with me and so she was shouting at me and saying as much.

Given that I'm usually the first one out of the house in the mornings, and so I will always place my bike, shoes and rucksack to facilitate my swift exit, and that, just before she headed out, I had warned her to be careful when walking down the stairs because of how my bike was parked, I had two choices when it came to how I should respond to my wife's anger at me:

a) I could apologise and promise that I'd be more careful parking my bike in future.

Vs.

b) I could deploy the "Well, I did just tell you to be careful..." line.

Not surprisingly, one of these would help to ease the situation (a), whereas the other would just exasperate matters (b). I'm embarrassed to say I went with option (b) because I had put my ego before my wife's feelings that, at that stressful moment, were more in need of soothing than they were of one-upmanship.

* * *

Why is it that divorce rates in the UK are so high?

I'd be willing to wager that one of the reasons is that many people don't realise that, as Stephen Covey elegantly describes in his book, *The seven habits of highly effective people*, LOVE IS A VERB; instead, many of us, as Hollywood movies intend us to, believe love to be a FEELING. The problem with feelings is that they are transient, i.e., they come and they go, and so many married couples will cite falling out of love as one of the main reasons for breaking up.

I'm not saying that love won't make you feel great when you find it because it does, and that's a good thing. I'm merely saying that love is a verb because it is something you do; something you actively need to work at to keep it alive. Such a proactive approach to love is far healthier in the longer term than the reactive person's approach to love where they are driven by emotions or feelings that may dissipate.

Ask anyone in a successful and loving relationship and they'll tell you it takes work. Ask a new-time parent that hasn't slept properly in weeks, and they'll say the same thing. And this is because love is something you do. It's about the sacrifices you make. Love is generated via loving actions.

* * *

If, for instance, you're in a non-ideal or an unfulfilling relationship, ask yourself the following question:

Am I proactively doing everything I can to make this relationship work or am I instead reactively focusing on, what I perceive to be, the other person's weaknesses?

You need to think really carefully before answering this question, because it is all too easy to point that accusing finger at the other person, to focus on the other person's flaws, the other person's shortcomings. And all too easy to not turn that accusing finger back in on yourself. Remember 'Shift your perspective' from Chapter 3? Well, you need to do that here and objectively try to see the other person's viewpoint. Is it possible that you are, at least partly, responsible for the relationship's stagnancy?

The following simple exercise may help you here:

Take a pen and paper and list all the things you are looking for as character traits in your ideal partner, be it, for instance, generosity, open-mindedness, patience and confidence. And then HONESTLY tick off all the things on your list you think best describe you too. This may help you to identify areas in need of self-improvement.

And if you were confiding your relationship woes to your personal journal, a close friend or a marriage counsellor, what kind of LANGUAGE would you use? Would it be reactive language, for instance:

"My wife makes me so angry."

Or

"If only my husband was more affectionate."?

If so, you are effectively transferring blame to the other person and absolving yourself of responsibility.

Instead, strive to take back some **RESPONSIBILITY** to make the relationship work.

When was the last time you brought her flowers?

When was the last time you decided to forgo that night out with your mates to spend a nice, romantic evening in with your partner where, shock horror, you even cooked them a nice meal?

ACTIVELY seek to love him or her. Try to be a better listener, be more patient, be more empathic and never take them for granted. For to do so, at the very least, you will have demonstrated to the other person you are investing into the relationship; that you are actively seeking to LOVE them.

And perhaps, in return, they may follow your example and seek to work at loving you back too.

Love is a verb.

* * *

That word "responsibility" keeps popping up, doesn't it?

This is no coincidence.

Once the dust settles, post-relationship, post-argument, post-conflict, other than in extreme cases (e.g. abusive partner), and once the emotion has all but dissipated, it's amazing how much more objective one can be in self-reflection. How much more honest one can be when it comes to identifying one's own contributions to a relationship or communication breakdown.

The key is trying to be that more objective version of yourself **NOW**. In that way, you may either sustain and build on what you already have or be much better prepared for the next time.

Good luck.

* * *

25. Love thy enemies

"The people for whom you least want to pray are the people for whom you most need to pray" - Criss Jami, poet and philosopher.

"Love thy enemies" or words to that effect are referenced several times in the Christian Bible, and there are various other versions of this statement knocking about in Zen and other philosophies.

Okay, it's been done to death, so why am I covering it in this book?

Because different people assign different meanings to this statement but many won't agree with it. And with good reason too. If someone has done you a serious wrong, why should you even like them, let alone love them? Surely self-preservation dictates that not only do you HATE your enemies, but you give them a wide birth also.

And this is what I would like to challenge here!

Now, our old buddy, Jordan Peterson, puts an interesting spin on it. He believes that genuine self-interest necessitates getting on with others because we are ALL CO-DEPENDENTS, even if they are our enemies. And that it may be the case that your enemies - let's say the school bully or that malevolent manager at work - are probably enduring their own form of hell. Maybe they are themselves at the receiving end of some kind of abuse or persecution out of their control.

So why should you add to this NEGATIVE DEFICIT when instead you can offer them compassion that may bring them back from the brink in some small way? And in doing so, this may make your life a little easier too, when they realise that you are not the problem here.

* * *

I genuinely believe that sometimes you can even kill them with kindness. Not literally, of course.

To a story that may help explain this:

A while back, my parents were starting up a new café in central London, and my friend and I were handing out promotional flyers outside of a nearby London underground train station. Some people took the flyers, others ignored us. I'll never forget this one time, though, a large and imposing guy coming up and standing toe-to-toe with me, snatching a flyer out of my hand and aggressively barking into my face:

"Why the fuck should I bother with one of these?!"

I softly replied (mostly because I was crapping myself) words to the effect of:

"Okay, sorry, no problem."

And amazingly, when he realised that I wasn't going to engage him at his level of aggression, he instantly switched. His shoulders dropped, and his gaze softened. His entire body language changed from Clubber Lang in Rocky 3 to Bill and Ted on a chill day.

In some kind of defeated way, he then said:

"Let me take some more (flyers) so that I can hand them out to my mates. We're working just around the corner."

And, a week later, when the café opened, he and his builder buddies dropped in every morning for the '£2.95 - Full English Breakfast plus cup of tea or coffee' promotional offer we were running. Yes, £2.95, it was that long ago!

Now this guy wasn't my enemy, not least of all because I didn't need to endure his moodiness regularly. The lesson I learnt here, though, was that I'm sure it wouldn't have turned out anywhere near as well for me had I matched his aggression.

Instead, I engaged him respectfully. I had shown him more compassion than he had shown me.

* * *

Let's get back to that school bully or nasty co-worker:

What if, again, we strive to shift perspective and seek to understand why they are the way they are. Had we been in their shoes, is it possible that we would have turned out the same way? Or maybe you can even find something about that person you can LOVE. Sure, they don't treat you well, but maybe they're a doting parent, or they volunteer at the local hospice. Or maybe you can kill them with kindness by smiling or doing something nice for them.

And even if all your efforts to love your enemies don't pay off, even if they don't become your friend or someone you can get along with, at least you will have found some inner peace by:

- accepting that some people just are the way they are;

- choosing to forgive and let go of past resentments or events that cannot be undone and understanding that there is no point holding on to them when all they will do is eat us up from the inside out.

***

It'll be useful to add something here that Jay Shetty once shared in an interview with Tom Bilyeau on the latter's podcast, Impact Theory, which I highly recommend, by the way.

Shetty said:

Just as there are people that you love and that don't love you back; there are people that invest in you, that love you and yet you don't love them in return.

Just think about that for a second, as it may not have occurred to you before.

Shetty believes that, as I touched on earlier in this book, whatever you put out into the world, you get back, including love. It's just that the love won't necessarily be coming back from the same people you love.

And it's the same with hurt.

You will have likely been hurt by people you never hurt - your supposed enemies; *yet you'll have likely done the same to others.*

Love thy enemies.

* * *

Did you find this chapter challenging?

Were there any principles you totes couldn't get on with?

I remember once being in church when the priest's homily covered the 'Love thy enemies' principle. He described how years before in theological college, a fellow rookie just couldn't get his head around the notion of loving his enemies and so he jumped ship.

I found this interesting because dogmas such as the Ten Commandments are founded on social scientific principles. It's as if some very forward-thinking social scientists and philosophers worked out how best we humans should interact with one another to keep the peace and advance the species. And so, it makes sense to me that, even though someone else may hate or work against you, you should never lower yourself to their level. Otherwise, the consequently hopeless world, now over-laden with feuding, self-interested and embittered humans, would self-destruct.

Instead, by demonstrating compassion, empathy and forgiveness, inner and outer peace is within reach.

The reason I focus on this principle in particular for Chapter 5's outro is because 'Love thy enemies' is the one that most of us (including a rookie priest!) would find to be the most challenging, as it stretches our better capacities to their very limits. And so, if you can get your head around the fact that you should still put the love out there anyway, even though it may not be reciprocated by its intended recipients, then surely everything else between is also possible.

And that, my friend, is when the magic happens.

* * *

CHAPTER 6

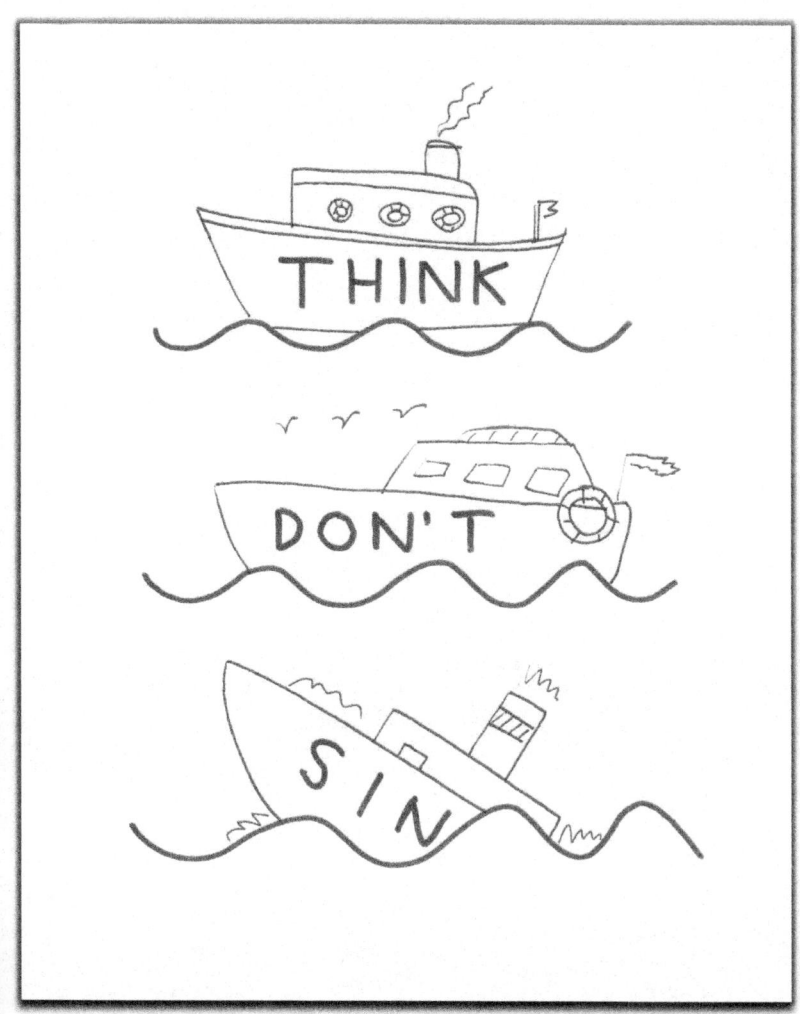

CHAPTER 6
ACCEPT REALITY

This chapter challenges the learned wisdom from earlier chapters.

For sometimes, shit happens that we just can't think our way out of.

26. Accept that which you cannot control

"Accept hardships as the path to peace" - Reinhold Niebuhr, theologian and ethicist.

I will start by telling you that the world owes you nothing.

That you are not special nor are you entitled to anything.

Fairness or karma is a social construct much like luck, justice or destiny.

The laws of nature or circumstance, much like the weather, do not much care for the laws of humans.

As famously quoted by Ben Shapiro, the controversial American political commentator:

"Facts do not care about your feelings."

Let's face it, life seems tough, brutal and unfair at times. Sometimes bad, real things will happen to good people. Things that cannot be undone by a positive mindset. Current US President, Joe Biden, is a case in point.

When Biden was 30 years old, he tragically lost his first wife and daughter in a car accident and, more recently, his son, Beau, died from cancer. Under such circumstances, many others would have felt embittered or self-pitying. Not Biden, though.

On his desk, the US president keeps a present that his father gave him shortly after the first tragedy: A rectangular frame with a cartoon in it. It depicts Hagar The Horrible being blasted in a boat by a storm and he shouts up to the heavens:

"Why me?!"

To which God replies:

"Why not (you)?"

Biden said of this during a conversation with a journalist[23]:

---

[23] Piers Morgan, CNN, 2015

"My dad was always saying to us when we were down about something, 'Where is it written that the world owes you a living, pal? Get up.' This cartoon was his way of saying there is no way to rationalise what has taken place. It can happen to anyone, at any time. But if you don't get up, it will crush you. I didn't fully appreciate the cartoon's message at the time, but it's become such a valuable one to me, especially after Beau died."

Biden then explained that it was his purpose, his Why, that helped him to get through these difficult times, his purpose being to help as many people as he can.

We explored 'purpose' earlier and 'managing adversity' is up next, so I won't dive into them here, but instead, I want to focus on **ACCEPTANCE**.

Acceptance is understanding that some things are simply out of our control. That no matter how proactive, successful or effective we are in other aspects of our lives, some things we just cannot change.

Acceptance doesn't mean being happy about something, nor does it mean forgetting it or pretending that something hasn't occurred or won't happen. Acceptance is embracing the present, good or bad, so you can shape the future. Acceptance moves you from a position of no control (of the cause) to one of control (of the effect). And just because something is out of our control, it doesn't mean we can't better prepare for it. As explorer and writer, Sir Rannulph Fiennes, once remarked:

There's no such thing as bad weather, just inappropriate clothing.

And he had a point. I can't control the wind or snow or rain, but I can better minimise its negative impact on my day by taking the appropriate measures: I can wear a raincoat, use an umbrella or take a bus to work as opposed to riding my bike.

Or, in anticipation of more stressful situations, I can work on building up my emotional resilience (next principle). At the end of each day, for instance, I can reflect on how my day went:

What went well for me?

What didn't go so well?

What can I learn to handle better in the future?

If a colleague shouts at me or I get a stinging email perhaps, as per 'Shift your perspective', I can try to see things from their viewpoint. In doing so, I may respond in a more mature and constructive manner. And, little by little, as I build up my emotional maturity, I am better placed to accept the more challenging or stressful situations that life will throw at me.

According to Richard Templar, when you come up against a major crisis that cannot be changed - death, divorce or a terminal diagnosis, for instance - you will need to be the one to adapt, you will need to be the one to change, and so building up your emotional resilience during the sunny days will better prepare you for winter. Again, you don't have to like it or want it. It is so tempting to fight it, refuse to believe it or try to change reality, however, you are just delaying the inevitable.

We can only begin to heal once we understand that the big stuff in life will change us. And we need to be willing to go through this process. That's what you're accepting: some things just are and you're the one that needs to change.

Templar observes that *ACCEPTANCE can usually be seen by an individual taking ownership for themselves and their actions:*

- These individuals begin to accept responsibility.

- They work towards accomplishing tasks and then are proud of the results.

- They are willing to change their behaviours in response to the needs of others.

- They are more content as they journey towards a more normalised life knowing that happiness and fulfilment will once again be within reach.

Accept that which you cannot control.

* * *

Not all things outside of our control are necessarily bad or negative.

When they are, though, that's when we need to have some powerful strategies up our sleeve.

27. Manage adversity

"Let me embrace thee, sour adversity, for wise men say it is the wisest course" - *William Shakespeare, playwright and poet.*

My dad passed away about 6 months ago (at the time of writing this principle) and I think I have only fairly recently got past the stage of shock. My dad was old, but unfortunately, his demise was brought about by the neglect and incompetence of the hospital supposed to be treating him which, as I'm sure you'll imagine, has exasperated matters no end.

It is only now that his passing is starting to land for me as the rest of the world has kind of gone back to normal, but now I more fully realise that he is no longer a part of it.

I've lost family and friends before but never an immediate family member, and so this is new territory for me as I have taken on a new level of grief I have never known.

You may imagine then that, with all the learnings I have undertaken, or the research I have done, leading to this book, the pain or grief process associated with loss is of particular interest. I hope that you can draw some use or comfort from this principle also.

I referenced Kain Ramsay's book, *Responsibility Rebellion,* earlier. In it, Ramsay says that we will ALL face adversity in our lives, be it through loss, poor health, job insecurity or financial jeopardy to name but a few. And it is difficult to channel positive thinking during such upsetting and frightening times, but the only beneficial response is to acknowledge your emotions, allow yourself to feel them, and then you move on.

Entirely focus on asking yourself constructive questions about what you're feeling and then work your way through and out of your situation.

Not easy.

Essentially though, one shouldn't wallow in the feeling nor allow one's mind to become consumed with helpless and destructive thoughts. Don't allow destructive thoughts to take up so much space in your head they become part of your identity. Don't allow adversity to become part of who you are, and don't become fond of it. Some people will even wear adversity as some badge of honour. They define their present and future selves by their emotional baggage. This isn't healthy.

Instead, adversity should be regarded as a challenge you are glad to accept and overcome.

This is where emotional intelligence or emotional quotient (EQ) comes in. According to helpguide.org[24], EQ is the ability to understand, use and manage your emotions in positive ways to relieve stress, communicate effectively, empathise with others, overcome challenges, and to defuse conflict.

As Ramsay points out, though, many people you encounter will, unfortunately, lack emotional intelligence.

Why?

Parents and educational establishments have a lot to answer for, actually. How common is it for children to be taught the value of emotions? Boys growing up in my generation during the 80s or 90s, for instance, were encouraged to not be 'cry babies'. Stiff upper lip 'n' all that.

---

[24] A website dedicated to improved mental health awareness.

And what do you think it is that leads children or even adults to become bullies? It is caused by insecurity due to lack of EQ because they just can't emotionally connect with others. Do you think, for instance, we'd be in the middle of a Russia-Ukraine conflict right now if certain people had more EQ?

With so little emotional intelligence out there, while it's tempting to stoop down and meet others where they're at, DON'T! It is of the upmost importance that you uphold your emotional intelligence standards at all times, lead others by example and wish the best for them.

Emotional intelligence is a delicate balance between rational thinking, emotional awareness, and expression, which requires continuous effort, practice and focus.

So, what can we do to build up our emotional intelligence skill set, which, by the way, and following on from the helpguide.org definition, may be defined by the following attributes?

Effective:

- Self-management;

- Self-awareness;

- Social-awareness;

And

- Good relationship management.

Answer:

- Acknowledge your emotion.

Don't bury it, don't hide it, don't deny it, don't be ashamed or embarrassed of it. Writing it down or journalling it may be useful here.

- Analyse your emotion.

Think about it. How and why does it make you feel the way you feel? Remember what I said earlier: Is your current emotional experience a reflection of your early life experience?

- Accept the emotion by considering differing perspectives.

For instance, I accept the grief for losing my dad because it acknowledges the great love and joy that having him in my life brought me. And you know what? It's well worth it. When you lose a loved one, the pain you feel may also offer you some comfort because it causes you to be *grateful* for and reflective of the time you had with that person when they were alive.

Grief means you had love in your life.

The key, though, as per 'Practice gratitude', is to try to be grateful whilst your loved ones are still alive in anticipation of the inevitable fact that nothing lasts forever.

Journaling again may be useful for some here as it allows psychological separation from one's emotions.

- Handle your emotion.

Read on the topic, learn about coping strategies, talk to friends that have themselves been through what you're going through: How did they deal with it?

- Practice self-care.

This includes going for walks or exercising, as this increases cerebral blood flow and so improves mental clarity and reduces ruminating thoughts. As per this book's first principle, healthy sleep is massively important, and breathing techniques and other grounding exercises are useful tools too that enable you to live in and acknowledge the moment, the Now, to take your mind away from the painful past or the anxious future (Chapter 7).

And finally

- Engage with others.

Strive to recognise their mainly non-verbal cues to help steer them through their own challenging emotions. For to do so, according to Ramsay, will not only bring you fulfilment, but you will find that others will regard you as reliable, trusting and inspirational.

* * *

Given the impact that death has on all of us, sooner or later, and given that everything we do in life is consciously or unconsciously linked to our fear of death, I feel I need to end this principle with another Mark Manson quote as it offers us all some beautiful and meaningful reassurance:

"...in a bizarre, backwards way, death is the light by which the shadow of all of life's meaning is measured. Without death, everything would feel inconsequential, all experience arbitrary, all metrics and values suddenly zero."

Manage Adversity.

* * *

This chapter's final principle is a deeper dive into a powerful coping strategy that has yet to be mentioned as it merits its own limelight.

28. Reframe with humour

"Humour is mankind's greatest blessing" – Mark Twain, writer and humourist (he would say that!)

As I said near the start of this chapter, it may sometimes feel like the universe is conspiring against us.

It rains when you don't have your umbrella, you miss your bus so you will be late for that meeting, you make up time by running to the office, only to find when you get there that your meeting was tomorrow morning instead!

You are soaked, tired, sweaty and your work colleagues are laughing at you. You have 3 choices:

- You can scream;

- You can be angry;

Or

- You can laugh at yourself too.

And, not surprisingly, laughing at yourself is best for your mental health, plus your work colleagues will like you much better for it too! This may not be easy at the time so perhaps you can imagine yourself relaying the experience to somebody else later on and making it as funny as you can:

"...and you'll never guess what happened when I got there..."

According to Richard Templar, one of the wonderful things about being human is that anecdotes about things going horribly wrong are a wonderful source of humour *after* the event.

The trick described in this principle, however, is not to wait until afterwards, but instead it's about using the prospect of 'cashing in' on the anecdote to help you *now*.

Whilst volunteering for a charity that helped people in distress, one thing Templar noticed was that even people going through the most dreadful traumas seemed to cope better when they laughed at themselves. And the reason he assigned to this was that, in order to laugh at themselves, they had to take a mental step back and view themselves from someone else's perspective. And it was this distance, this almost objective self-observation, that seemed to give them the detachment they needed to cope with their situation.

They were essentially reframing their situation.

Following on from what was said in 'Accept that which you cannot control,' humour may well be one of the most powerful weapons in your armoury when it comes to acceptance.

Laughing in general is great at reducing stress and improving mental health.

* * *

A story:

When I was at UCL, one of my lecturers had a really annoying habit of snorting or, to be a little more descriptive, blowing his nose from the inside and swallowing it! All the bloody time!

(Enjoy your lunch)

At first, I found this greatly distracting and I just couldn't concentrate on his teachings. This was stressful because I needed to pass his exams.

It was only after I moaned about it to some classmates, did we create a game whereby essentially, at every one of this lecturer's classes, we would keep a running tally of how many snorts he would blurt out. We turned it into a bit of light-hearted fun, whereby every week we would see if he could beat his own record! And snortly thereafter, I had become completely oblivious to his annoying habit because I had made light of it. I had deflected it away from my stress sensors by using humour to reframe it.

You may apply humour to many situations where you need to spend time with patronising or annoying work colleagues or relatives, for instance, perhaps by comparing funny notes with others that also need to suffer these people.

And finally, I find humour to be of some comfort with grief. Sometimes I'll be chatting to my mum about my late dad, and we'll remember something he did or said that was funny, and so we'll laugh about it, and, in that moment, our grief will become a beautiful, shared memory that we can both reflect on with fondness and joy. And we'll remember how lucky we are to have had him in our lives.

Reframe with humour.

* * *

SUMMARY:

And so, as we start to come around full circle, it is worth recapping what we have covered so far, before leaving you with the final chapter 7, that considers how best to understand and use our most valuable and finite commodity.

Until now, we have looked at six core areas:

Chapter 1 - First, let's get our house in order - laid down a solid foundation with some common sense principles that provided the springboard from which the remaining principles of this book would emerge in all their glory.

For unless we will take some simple steps to look after our bodies and our minds by:

- Striving to get some decent sleep;

- Purging our minds of unhealthy obstacles or distractions;

- Relying less on digital devices that are dumbing us down or overloading us and causing anxiety;

- Saying 'no' to the things that would otherwise overburden us, burn us out or undermine our authenticity,

...then what chance will we have to turn up and be ready to play our 'A' game? Our 'A' game being to deploy the remaining principles of this book to overcome life's various challenges.

Answer:

Much less of a chance.

* * *

Chapter 2 - Know thy self - will have got you to dig deep by challenging everything you assume you know about yourself or the world around you, by asking you some frank questions. For instance:

- Are you authentic and dependable?

- Are you open to external feedback?

- Are you willing and able to challenge your limiting beliefs?

Acknowledge all of those areas of your life you are doing well in, while simultaneously seeking and working on those areas in need of improvement or overhaul. The latter will require you to accept:

You don't know what you don't know.

By incorporating these principles into your life, you have every chance of coming out the other side a more reliable, self-aware and better-rounded person.

* * *

Chapter 3 – Are you positive? - will have focused on the significant benefits of:

- Broader perspective consideration and patience;

- Affirming self-talk and signalling;

- Taking full responsibility and not being a complainer;

- A positivity bias;

- Regularly practising gratitude,

...and how to apply these principles to your life.

I cannot overstate the wondrous impact on both physical and mental health that a more positive outlook brings with it.

Inward and outward compassion is key.

Mindset is everything.

* * *

Chapter 4 -What actually matters? - should have got you to ask yourself some pretty fundamental questions such as:

- What is it that drives you?

- What does a fulfilled life look like to you?

- How would you like to be remembered long after you are gone?

Please spend some time reflecting on these principles, my friend, as the answers you come up will tell you whether the life you are living now is aligned with your purpose.

And if it isn't:

What steps can you take to address this?

This is proper shit so please don't dilly-dally or put it off, as you would short-change yourself and those closest to you.

As much as you can, everything you do should either be fulfilling to you right now or, at the very least, be taking you closer to your most fulfilling outcomes.

* * *

Chapter 5 - Connection, connection, connection – looks more outwardly still, as it tips its hat to the power of social interactions - a major contributor to personal wellbeing.

Despite our complexities, egos and sensibilities, we are social animals that benefit from both the application and receipt of some basic 'human' principles. These range from fundamentals such as:

- Being genuinely appreciative;

- Remembering names;

Through

- Creating a proactive gap between stimulus and response;

- Genuinely listening and not preaching;

To

- Loving both those closest to you and your enemies.

Empathy, patience and appreciation are very much starter, main course and dessert should you wish to thrive in your social interactions and get back as much as you put out. And then some.

* * *

Chapter 6 - Accept reality - deals with life's harsher realities that will challenge much of the preceding chapters and describes acceptance, management and reframing strategies to better understand, cope with and overcome:

- All we cannot control;

- Adversity.

Acceptance is the first step in overcoming any challenging situation, then responsibility and persistence of strategy.

Life is tough at times for all of us, but you can overcome anything it throws at you, should you choose to.

* * *

And so, to the big finish...

CHAPTER 7

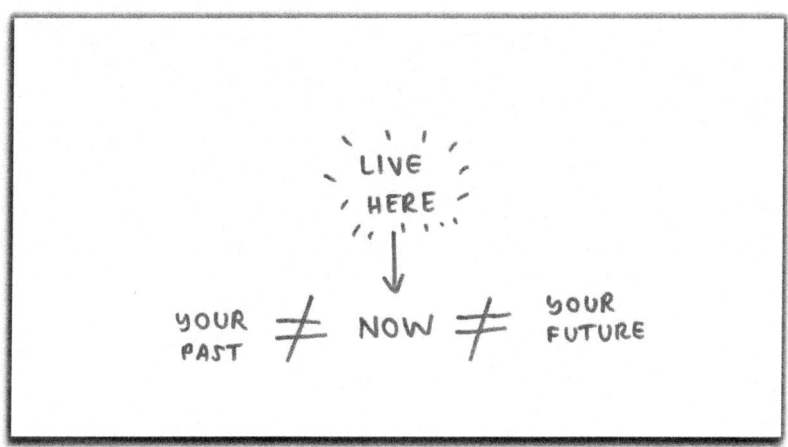

CHAPTER 7
Tick Tock
(No, the other one)

29. Live in the Now

"The best preparation for the future is to live as if there were none"
– Albert Einstein, theoretical physicist.

Why are some people thrill-seekers?

They'll race cars, they'll jump out of planes, they'll free-climb mountains or skyscrapers. Why do people get a buzz from doing these dangerous things?

Let us understand why without going into the physiochemistry of it all:

It's because they are forced into the **NOW**. Into the **PRESENT**.

According to Eckhart Tolle in his book, *The power of Now*, for those few moments, thrill-seekers are intensely alive and experiencing a state free of time, of problems, of the burden of personality, and free of thinking. Otherwise, slipping away from the present moment, even for a split second, may mean death.

Think about that for a moment.

In those exhilarating moments, you do not have time to even *think*. Call it instinct, call it muscle memory, call it whatever you want, it just kicks in.

* * *

Now, psychological fear comes in many forms such as worry, anxiety, dread or phobia. Psychological fear is always of something that might happen in the future; not of something happening now. Essentially you are in the here and now, while your mind is in the future. This creates an 'anxiety gap', even though technically, the only thing that is real is **NOW**; not the future because it hasn't happened yet.

So, there's an anxiety gap between the real now and the mind projection that is the **FUTURE**.

Similarly, the **PAST** no longer exists. There are things that happened in the past that we can learn from, which is very important of course, but we may also derive negative emotions from the past. This may be anger or irritation at what someone has said or done, or perhaps frustration at not having got that promotion at work.

One drawback of our minds is therefore that many of us spend inordinate amounts of **THINKING TIME** dwelling on the past or worrying about the future; neither of which is real because neither of which is now.

Have I lost you yet? I hope not! :)

* * *

Tolle is not saying that considering the past, or planning for the future, are not useful things to do when one has lessons to learn, losses to process or practical matters to organise. However, our minds are intrinsically linked to TIME.

The compulsion is to live almost exclusively through memory and anticipation. Thus, creating an endless preoccupation with past and future, and an unwillingness to honour and acknowledge the present moment and allow it to be.

In Tolle's own words:

The compulsion arises because the past gives you an identity and the future holds the promise of salvation, of fulfilment in whatever form. Both are illusions.

Acknowledge the present moment and allow it to be because it is impossible to experience, do, think or feel anything outside of the now.

What simple things can we do to be more in the present and reduce the impact of negative emotions anchored to the past and/or future?

- Focused breathing.

A friend once taught me the '4:6 breathing technique', designed to reduce anxiety and induce a state of calm, which is particularly useful when entering into more stressful environments, for instance, when giving a presentation. You breathe in slowly for 4 seconds and then out again, but even more slowly, for 6 seconds, and then repeat for anything between 1 to 10 minutes a day. There are many variations on this technique, the key being to make your exhalations longer and slower than your inhalations and simply counting the seconds.

Such breathing techniques are widely acknowledged to encourage the body's more relaxed 'rest and digest' (parasympathetic) state versus its more stressed 'fight or flight' (sympathetic) state. Endurance athlete, Christopher Bergland, says these techniques will increase heart rate variability associated with "lower chronic stress levels, better overall health and improved cognition."

First thing in the morning and before breakfast, I will sit in my kitchen, close my eyes and spend 5 to 10 minutes focusing in on my 4:6 breathing and then on the sounds of my 'Now' surroundings. An airplane passing by in the distant skies perhaps or my refrigerator that sounds like some 'crazy noises jukebox'. I will push myself to keep my mind focused only on those things.

There are numerous breathing and meditation techniques out there that you may want to explore and see what best works for you. I'd recommend keeping it simple though if you're starting out.

- Making time for basic pleasures.

Going for walks or smelling flowers in your garden or park, for instance, are good grounding exercises. Or merely appreciating the beauty and wonder in simple things, maybe your curtains or a chair, anything.

Or the next time you're eating a meal, take a few moments to really think about that meal. How it looks, tastes, smells. The 'how' is more important than the 'what.'

For in doing these individual things, you may experience the Now because you are not thinking about anything else outside of that thing in that moment. As I'll touch on again later, multi-tasking is a myth and so serves us particularly well here as you will only ever be able to truly focus on the one thing.

- Another useful grounding strategy, often used to help people overcome panic attacks, for instance, is finding somewhere comfortable to sit and then, wherever you are, focusing on:

* 5 x things you can see;

* 4 x things you can feel (for instance, the fabric of your skirt);

* 3 x things you can hear;

* 2 x things you can taste;

* 1 x thing you can smell.

And then take a few slow and deep breaths.

Grounded yet? Good!

It'll be challenging initially to do these grounding exercises if there's already stress or distraction buzzing about in your head but, with repetition and practice, it'll get easier and easier to do, and eventually you'll be able to use these habits to help block out unwanted, negative emotions. And I would strongly recommend continuing to do these exercises, even when everything's peachy, as you'll then be better equipped for those not-so-good days.

The power of Now explicitly states that - while the brain is, for lack of a better description, a highly developed tool - by better connecting to the Now, one may significantly reduce the pain, stress and anxiety associated with a 'chattering mind.' Therefore, one will have a greater clarity of thought when it is needed!

Live in the now.

* * *

The only way that one may reconcile the 'Now' principle just gone with the 'Time' principle to come is to remember that the past is a collection of 'Now' moments that have already occurred whilst the future is a collection of 'Now' moments that have yet to happen. Otherwise, it may seem that we are understating the importance of time.

30. Use your time well

"Time isn't the main thing. It's the only thing" - Miles Davis, jazz musician.

Steven Bartlett, star of television series, Dragons Den UK, and podcast, Diary of a CEO, has an interesting way of allocating his time to things that may also enable you to better prioritise the more important things in your life.

Bartlett will essentially treat the hours in his day as casino chips. Hence, there's 24 chips each day. The returns - or the quality of life you get - are based on how you place your chips on the metaphorical roulette table. For instance, you use 8 chips on sleep and so you are left with 16 chips. You might then, for instance, commit 2 chips to connections with family and friends, 9 chips go on work, 3 chips go on checking your smartphone and watching television, 1 chip goes on walking your dog or spending time in nature, and so on.

...and the roulette wheel of life keeps spinning. And it shows you the return on your chips. This is deciding your life.

The only thing we have control of in our life, the only thing within the centre-point of our influence, is how we use these chips. There is no other 'real' currency in life other than these chips.

And, unlike other forms of currency, once time has been spent, you cannot get it back.

And yet, without going into Stephen Hawking's[25] territory, time is merely a human construct we use to measure out, make sense of, or organise the world or universe around us. Time enables us to calculate with a high degree of accuracy when we are likely to see Halley's Comet again[26], or when I need to take a taxi to the airport to make my flight.

Anyway, you will need to play these finite chips as well as you can in order to live your best, most fulfilling life!

* * *

---

[25] Theoretical physicist, author and brainiac extraordinaire.
[26] If you're fussed, 2061 AD: every 76 years.

In all the life coaching, investment and entrepreneur type training courses or presentations that I've consumed, the one thing that ALL ultra-successful people will agree on is that TIME is our most precious commodity.

And so, like the ultra-successful, you will need to consider your opportunity costs.

This means that whenever you play your chips or invest time in a particular activity, this comes at the expense of something else, of some other opportunity. You cannot play both football and tennis at the same time, next Monday night at 7 o'clock. If you play tennis, then that comes at the expense of not playing football, or, if you take on a full-time 5-year postgraduate medical degree, you will unlikely be able to also do a full-time history degree, travel the world for 12 months or become a full-time cast member of Coronation Street.

Opportunity costs.

* * *

So, what is important to you?

Ignoring everything else that has happened in your life up until this moment, what is important to you in going forward now?

How best should you spend your time?

We are all different and so we have differing priorities. Maybe you have kids, maybe you don't have kids, maybe you've retired from your job or maybe you're just starting out in a new career. With so many options, choices or opportunities out there, how do we optimise our use of time for the maximum return?

Chris Bailey, productivity guru and author of articles in lifehack.org, proposes several simple ways for us to make the most of our time:

- Slow down.

While this may sound counterintuitive, Bailey says that when you slow things down, what you actually do becomes more meaningful.

For instance, you can drive through a beautiful forest in your car, listening to the radio and whilst chatting to your mate in the passenger seat and then, without even realising it, you're out of the forest and it's like you were never there. Walk through the forest alone, however, and you better take in its beauty, sounds and smells without distraction, and so what you were doing became more meaningful.

Slowing down brings more meaning to how you spend your time, be it going for a walk, playing a guitar, reading a book or spending time with a loved one. You are 'living in the Now' (previous principle).

- Structure your free time.

According to Mihaly Csikszentmihalyi (no, I can't pronounce it either), in his book, *Flow*, midday Sunday is "the unhappiest hour in America" because that's when people are the least productive. He argues that when we don't structure our time, we ruminate or do more pointless stuff. Structuring, even your free time, is proven to make you more motivated, focused and, ultimately, happier because it gives you direction and purpose.

- Do less.

When you do fewer things, you spread your time over less, and so you have much more of yourself to give to the things that you do do[27]. This enables you to do these things better and so you will feel more productive.

- Prioritise the things that matter most.

Tying into the idea of doing fewer things, Bailey believes that the best way to make sure you get the most out of your time is to start with what matters the most to you and work backwards from there to the things that matter least.

I'll add a caveat here: The conscious part of our human brains can only focus on one thing at any one time. For instance, no one can drive a car safely whilst having a virtual meeting on their smartphone. Multi-tasking is a myth. Instead, we switch our attention from task to

---

[27] ffs!

task extremely quickly, coming at the detriment of the original task which, should we return to later on, will take much longer to get back into. Aka, focus only on your immediate priorities!

And finally,

- Think about how quickly you use up your chips.

Appreciating just how little time you have will help you put that time to better use. One trick I'd suggest here is to consider that, while you use money to *buy* things, time is what you use to *pay* for things. For instance, if you earn £20 per hour, a £60 pair of shoes will cost you three hours of your life.

Please do not waste those precious chips of yours on things that don't matter!

Savour each moment as if it were your last. For you just don't know when that last moment is.

Use your time well.

* * *

OUTRO

So here we are.

I didn't expect to find you here quite so soon, but anyway, make yourself comfortable.

Cup of tea?

I thought long and hard about how I should end this book as I wanted it to be memorable for you.

Then I remembered that, not least of all because this book is so easy to follow (I think), its principles merit re-visiting sometimes, either as a quick refresher for those ones you have adopted, or as a way for you to identify a new principle you have yet to take out for a spin. And so, I'm hoping that you will come to regard this book as an old friend. A wise old timer you can lean on anytime you need some re-calibration.

This has kind of taken the pressure off of my 'big finish' because there's not much more wisdom lurking beyond this point. Actually, there is, so please keep reading!

I'm sorry that I included some swear words in this book and I hope that these didn't offend you in any way. It's just that I don't give a fuck. Shift your perspective. Wherever swear words are deployed, I feel they lend the text the intended passion and weight of feeling.

* * *

To get this back on track...you may have noticed that Chapter 1 began with 'Invest in your sleep' while the final Chapter 7 has just concluded with 'Use your time well.'

This was by design.

I cannot over-stress how fundamental to your mental health and wellbeing decent sleep is. It is the foundation upon which all the other principles here are built. For a well-rested body and mind is better able to function, and thus better able to deploy the box of tricks described within this book.

And time is our most valuable commodity, and it is so very important that you use it well and to your advantage. When you're on your death bed, you will likely be your most authentic self ever. And what is it that EVERYONE on their death bed (that isn't a miserable fucker) will want more than anything else in the world?

Well, it won't be more money, a better social life or the latest iPhone. They will want more TIME.

If you intend to incorporate any of The Much Better You's principles into your own life, I'd say these two are fairly good starting points, while everything else in between is massively important also.

Yes, yes, nearly done...

When cycling to work, I once noticed how a fellow cyclist in front of me had well-developed calf muscles (no, I'm not a weirdo). This likely meant that he regularly cycled to work, and so I reflected on how his fitness was a welcome by product of his commute to work. So essentially in doing one useful thing (commuting), another useful thing came crashing out (fitness and likely better mental and physical health).

And this reflects life more generally, in that the more 'good stuff' you do, often the better other things in your life will become also. The more you read, the smarter you will inevitably be. The better your quality of sleep or exercise, the better your mental health or the more manageable your stress levels. The more gratitude you have generally, the happier and more fulfilled your life will be.

What I'm trying to say is that, while this book is far from an exhaustive list of mental health and wellbeing lifehacks, by engaging with its principles, the benefits will be far wider reaching than you will ever possibly imagine.

* * *

And now for the proper finish...

One common thread that ties all these chapters and their principles together is that one shouldn't need to rely on other people's behaviours or actions, nor on external events, to determine one's own responses or actions.

Successful people, and I mean in all aspects of their lives, are willing to do the things that unsuccessful people don't want to do.

Take responsibility for all areas of your life within your control and determine your own outcomes.

Thank you so much for reading this book.

I very much hope that you enjoyed reading it and found some use within its pages and perhaps some comfort too.

If not, tough tits, give this copy to your enemies. For the greatest fulfilment in life comes from serving others.

* * *

CLOSING THOUGHT

In the last few years of my dad's life, he fought with heart disease and depression, most especially during the Covid lockdowns that saw his daily routine come grinding to a halt. Despite this, his compassion, love, sense of humour and character remained fully intact.

We shared some wonderful moments in the last few months of his life. I'll never forget how this one night, to give my mum a bit of a break, I slept in my parents' bedroom to help monitor and assist my dad, as he usually had to get up during the night. As I often liked to do, and as I found that it momentarily distracted him from his woes, I would ask my dad to tell me about his adventures as a boy growing up in the mountains of Tuscany. Given that he grew up in a remote village during the Second World War occupied by the Nazis, you may imagine how fascinating his stories were. Another book for another time perhaps.

But that night he recounted for me one of his earliest living memories. A time when he was lying in his bed, in the house he was born in, and looking out of his bedroom window. He saw snow falling heavily on to the roof of the house opposite and he wondered to himself how on earth that roof was able to sustain the significant weight of the settling snow.

I'll never forget how my dad described this. It was as if he was a little boy again, so full of life and wonder. It was as if he was seeing it all again but for the first time.

Now I have visited my dad's old house in Italy and so I can imagine everything that he saw. Every detail, including the snow-laden roof of the house opposite.

I mention this here for two reasons: Firstly, this story holds a special memory for me, and I fear that I may never get around to recording it again, if not in this book; and secondly, because this roof reminded me of my dad towards the end of his life. Burdened with the weight of his thoughts and anxieties. I wished at the time that I could somehow melt the snow to take away some of the weight, but I couldn't.

I hope, however, that this book will help to melt some of that snow for you if you need it.

THE END

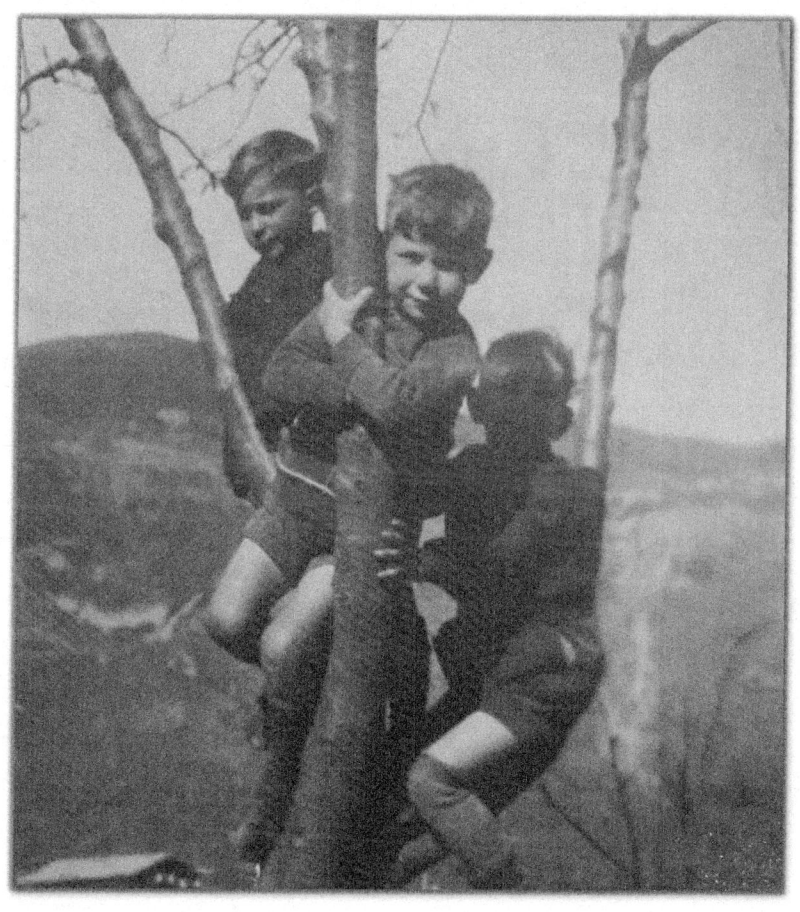

CLOSING THOUGHT

: ACKNOWLEDGMENTS

ACKNOWLEDGEMENTS

Without my mum, Brigida, dad, Ranieri, and wife, Sila, none of this would have been possible:

My mum and dad for their immense love and support throughout my life and for the endless opportunities they have brought me.

Sila, for her love, inspiration and ideas (many of which found their way into this book), editing skills and for her continuously pushing me to be my best self.

Thank you.

Enjoyed this book?

Go to TheMuchBetterYou.com and check out the surrounding shizzle!

Please leave this book a fabulous review and rating on Amazon to help raise its profile, sell more copies, make me rich and famous, and donate more money to MIND.

Please check out 'The 3 in 15 Podcast', FREE and available to listen to/download on all major platforms, inc. Apple, Amazon, Spotify and so forth.

And finally, if you like the music associated with 'The 3 in 15 Podcast' check out 'Leika' on Amazon Music, Spotify or iTunes, or www.soundcloud.com/LEIKA-the-BAND where you can download some of it for FREE.

Resources

Many wonderful resources were referenced in this book that enabled me to bring the best wellbeing and mental health awareness research to your attention. I wholeheartedly recommend that you explore the people/books/websites/podcasts.

Most chapter standalone quotes and all footnotes are not included here.

Chapter 1

- *"Say 'no' more" from 'Nudge, nudge' sketch, Monty Python*
- *Matthew WALKER, sleep scientist*
- *Jordan PETERSON, clinical psychologist and author*
- *Marie KONDO – 'The life changing magic of tidying up'*
- *VeryWellMind.com*
- *Jim KWIK, memory coach and author*
- *Jay SHETTY, life coach and author*
- *Nicole WASHINGTON, psychiatrist*
- *PsychCentral.com*
- *Inc.com*

Chapter 2

- *Stephen COVEY, 'The Seven habits of highly effective people'*

- Erich FROMM, social psychologist
- Mark MANSON, 'The subtle art of not giving a fuck'
- Richard TEMPLAR, 'The rules of living well'
- Jordan PETERSON, 'Twelve rules for life'
- MarkMANSON.net
- Kain RAMSAY, 'Responsibility Rebellion'

Chapter 3

- Stephen COVEY, 'The Seven habits of highly effective people'
- T. Harv EKER – 'Secrets of the millionaire mind'
- Gary VEE – entrepreneur and podcaster
- Jim KWIK
- Kazimierz DABROWSKI, psychologist
- Simon SINEK, author and speaker
- Kain RAMSAY, author and psychologist
- VeryWellMind.com
- Jim ROHN, motivational speaker

Chapter 4

- Stephen COVEY, author and speaker
- Simon SINEK, 'Start with why'

Chapter 5

- Dale CARNEGIE, 'How to win friends and influence people'
- Sigmund FREUD, founder of psychoanalysis
- Charles SCHWAB, steel magnate
- Viktor FRANKL, psychiatrist
- Jim KWIK, 'Kwik Brain' podcast
- Kristen FULLER, physician and author
- Stephen COVEY, 'The Seven habits of highly effective people'
- Jordan PETERSON
- Jay SHETTY
- Tom BILYEAU, 'Impact Theory' podcast

Chapter 6

- Joe BIDEN, current (2023) US President
- Richard TEMPLAR, author
- Kain RAMSAY, 'Responsibility rebellion'
- Rannulph FIENNES, explorer and writer
- HelpGuide.org
- Mark MANSON, blogger and author

Chapter 7

- Eckhart TOLLE, 'The power of Now'

- *Steven BARTLETT, entrepreneur and 'Diary of a CEO' podcast*
- *Chris BAILEY, productivity guru and author*
- *Mihaly CSIKSZENTMIHALYI, 'Flow'*
- *Christopher BERGLAND, Endurance athlete*

CRAZY PROMO OFFER

If you liked the chapter sketch designs, you can buy some as T-shirts or mugs by visiting TheMuchBetterYou.com and following the links therein.

TYPE in PROMO code TMBY25 to get 25% off the price.

Okay, I really am done now!

The Much Better You

Your wellbeing and mental health sorted

Dr Romano Giorgi

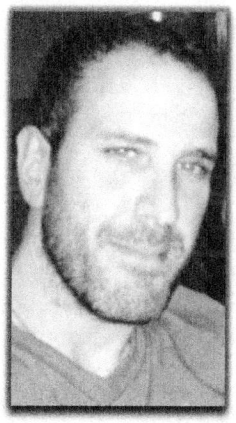

Printed in Great Britain
by Amazon